New

# The
# Thorn
# *in the*
# Starfish

W · W · NORTON & COMPANY

NEW YORK
LONDON

# *The* Thorn *in the* Starfish

*How the Human Immune System Works*

Robert S. Desowitz

FIRST EDITION

The text of this book is composed in Caledonia, with display type set in Baskerville. Composition and manufacturing by the Maple Vail Book Manufacturing Group. Book design by Marjorie J. Flock.

Library of Congress Cataloging-in-Publication Data

Desowitz, Robert S.
  The thorn in the starfish.

  Includes index.
  1. Immunology—Popular works.   I. Title.
QR181.7.D47   1987      616.07′9      86–23675

ISBN 0-393-02435-0

W. W. Norton & Company, Inc., 500 Fifth Avenue, New York, N.Y. 10110
W. W. Norton & Company Ltd., 37 Great Russell Street, London WC1B 3NU

1 2 3 4 5 6 7 8 9 0

*For* Carrolee

# Contents

# I

## *Historical Curtain Raisers*

# II

## *The Owner's Manual on the
Immune System*

# III

## *The Immune System in Sickness and in Health*

# IV

## *The Future of Immunity and Immunity in Your Future*

# Acknowledgments

I BEGAN this book during an incomparable month at the Rockefeller Study Center, the Villa Seberlloni in Bellagio, Italy. I am grateful to the Rockefeller Foundation for a scholar-in-residence award that allowed me to contemplate, in the most splendid and gracious of settings, the scope of the book and draft its opening chapters.

Nonscientist reviewers are essential when writing a "public" book on a scientific subject. I am indebted to Taylor A. Pryor and my wife, Carrolee (a nonscientist if there ever was one) for their patience and clear criticisms in reading copy, after copy, of the manuscript.

I am equally indebted to my scientist reviewers, Dr. Louis H. Miller of the National Institutes of Health, Dr. Richard B. Raybourne of the U.S. Food and Drug Administration, and Dr. Peter Kunstadter, for their time and effort in helping me keep the text accurate and readable.

I wish to thank Dr. Steven J. Berman for his advice on infectious diseases and, especially, for his many years of friendship.

Finally, I wish to express my appreciation to my editor, Ed Barber, vice president of W. W. Norton & Company, whose encouragement and advice have made this book possible.

ROBERT S. DESOWITZ

*The*
Thorn
*in the*
Starfish

# Preface: Immunity—
# More than a Shot in the Arm

LIKE MOST of you, I had my first lesson in basic immunology when I was about five years old. In the company of equally apprehensive peers I was taken into a room where a strange man mumbled a few incomprehensible words and suddenly stuck a large needle into my upper arm. There followed a swingeing pain and a wide-eyed howl. Some thirty years later my son had *his* first lesson in immunology. Being made of sterner stuff, in postinoculation indignation he administered a kick to the physician's shin. Not long ago in a small Bangladesh village I observed a similar collection of children who were about to be given that primary immunology lesson. They were of browner skin and darker eye than my group of Bronx trogs but equally terrified.

Thus, throughout the world immunology has been associated with "shots" against a constantly expanding variety of infectious diseases,[1] such as diphtheria, pertussis (whooping cough), yellow fever, poliomyelitis, tetanus, smallpox, measles, and rubella (German measles).

1. Infectious diseases are illnesses caused by pathogenic organisms, e.g., viruses, bacteria, and parasitic protozoa. However, disease (illness) is not the inevitable companion of infection. There are conditions in which the individual is *infected* with the microorganism but does not become ill. Immunity plays a major role in "dampening" the microbe—and that's what this book is largely about.

Immunization is still the major practical product of the science called *immunology*. It is a science that has provided humans and their domestic animals with an array of splendid triumphs over disease, most recently the final eradication of smallpox. Never again will there be deaths from this savage viral disease. Nor will we see those pockmarked faces in what was the disease's last great respository, the cities and villages of the tropics. Through a well-planned immunization campaign the smallpox virus has been exterminated in a few short years with the same irreversible absoluteness as the dodo, the carrier pigeon, and the Irish elk. The measles virus may be the next to go. Meanwhile, on the horizon of inventive expectation are vaccines to protect against hepatitis, herpes, AIDS virus, malaria, and in distant hope against some forms of cancer. Vaccines are of obvious importance in protecting our health but, in a sense, we are being immunized each day of our lives through contact with such alien substances as pathogenic (disease-causing) microbes, nonpathogenic microbes such as those that naturally colonize our gut and skin, environmental particulate matter, and even certain foods.

Under normal circumstances the immune system is the body's doctor, our personal physician that cures and protects us from a panoply of diseases. No drug is yet known, for example, to cure the common cold. The immune system alone effects recovery. We recognize this by attributing a contracted or prolonged illness to a state of "low resistance." That "resistance" is a pseudonym for immunity. Some people regard "resistance" as a personal property to be developed by a body building through strategies that include diet, meditation, exercise, and vitamins. This kind of "body building" is one of the few ways we have of controlling our lives in an untrammeled fashion. It also gives us escape from the medical establishment. All well and good, but if we and our immune system are to be our own physicians, we must apply the same rational management as the M. D. Self-treatment should be no less in quality and rationality than the prescription of our physician. Anything else is self-imposed quackery. Happily, we live in an Age of Information. The findings of biomedical research are no longer the exclusive property of our society's medicine men. Scientists—good scientists—now make every effort to explain their findings to the public.

Also happily, we live in the Golden Age of Immunology. Contemporary research has revealed the functions and expressions of immunity to be much more than a simple shot in the arm. The workings of the immune system have been found to be an incredible complex of interactions between specialized cells, tissues, and fluid factors of the body. The vanguard of immunological research has begun to discover how the immune system may be tuned, modulated, and its faulty parts replaced in ways that would astonish a Ferrari mechanic. Virtually every month there are reports in the biomedical journals of new drugs, diets, and biological agents that can be applied to manipulate the immune response. Also along the advancing research frontier is the exciting new work on the relationship of genetic inheritance and the character of the immune response of different individuals. And there are great expectations from the recently consumated marriage of genetic engineering and immunology.

In a better ordered world life and immunity would be consistently perfect. Such is not our world, however, and modern research has revealed immunity to have a darker side. Humans get no warranty when they are born. There are no recalls, no free replacement of parts if we come off the biological assembly line with a missing or faulty element of the immunological apparatus. Even given a normally competent immune system, there are certain nutritional, environmental, and microbial / parasitic pathogens that can cause a suppression and / or disarray to the immune response. In certain states, the immune system can faithlessly turn upon the body it is charged to protect or fail to response to the challenge of the invading pathogen. AIDS (acquired immunodeficiency syndrome) is the most notable example, although other, less publicized immunodeficiency states are equally dire. Hypersensitivity (allergic) states, which include asthma, are another example of immunity's darker side. And getting old doesn't help— the immune system accompanies the rest of the body on its march to senility.

I received my doctorate some three decades ago ("three decades" sounds less depressing than "thirty years") and I knew *everything*. Knowing everything goes with youth and the doctorate. However, with the passing years, despite reading, research, and efforts by my graduate students to keep the "old man" modern, it has become more and more difficult for me to maintain a good comprehension of how the immune system works. It seemed to me that if a biomedical scientist like myself was becoming confused by the complexity of modern immunology, what must be the level of public understanding? It's not that the immune system doesn't get a "good press." The immune system is currently news, but the explanations are mostly simplistic and, in their way, as confusing as a technical paper in the *Journal of Immunology*. And so this book—to present an explanation of how the immune system works in health and sickness, the strategies we might use to get the best from our immune system, and what we might expect from immunological research.

Unfortunately the immune system is so intricately complex that no explanation can be completely "without tears." There is, however, a fascination in that very complexity of interactions. Sudden immersion is uncomfortable, whether in cold oceans or unfamiliar bodies of knowledge, and for the sake of gradualism the book begins with the historical foundations of immunology. Also, you may find, as I have, the personalities of the Fathers of Immunology—Jenner, Pasteur, Metchnikoff, and Ehrlich—as intriguing as their discoveries. After the first four chapters there follow three chapters on the modern concepts of immunology. These are followed by chapters dealing with altered states of immunity, how these conditions arise, and how they may be controlled or the immune response augmented for our benefit. Finally, there is a section on the future of immunology.

I have tried to make our journey through the Immune Lands a pleasurable, understandable, and instructive experience. I hope I have succeeded. Clarity is not always easy for scientists-turned-writers, and intelligent lay readers would never tolerate the elliptical prose and conceptual obfuscations of scientific communication. My demurrer done, let us turn to Dr. Jenner's pretty, poxy milkmaids.

# I

*Historical Curtain Raisers*

# Chapter 1

# Dr. Jenner's Pretty, Poxy Milkmaids: Immunization's Opening Shots

THERE WERE no medical schools in Edward Jenner's England of the late eighteenth century. Medical training was by apprenticeship, and Jenner had the great good fortune to come under the tutelage of the greatest surgeon-anatomist of that time, John Hunter. In 1773, Jenner completed his training. Armed with knowledge of where most of the parts of the body were located (but, for many parts, a vague and often inaccurate idea of their function), of how to set broken bones, to "cut for the stone," to let blood to redress the humors, and of the rather exotic pharmacology of that era, Jenner returned to his home in Berkeley, Gloucestershire, to begin a medical practice. He also became John Hunter's naturalist–"leg man" in the country. The eclectic Hunter requested that Jenner collect and dispatch to London such rustic treasures as cuckoo eggs and hedgehogs. Jenner shared Hunter's love of natural history. As a bit of nonimmunological trivia we might note that Jenner was the first to describe the cruel primogeniture of the cuckoo, whereby the first to hatch pushed his

siblings out of the nest, and to their death, as they emerged
from their eggs.

In the eighteenth century, the long-held belief of the
causation of disease by magical and / or divine sources was
falling to reason and to science. Jenner regarded himself as
a part of the new wave, as a scientist in the "age of scientific
investigation," but nevertheless his ideas on the causes of
disease were tinged with Old Testament morality and belief.
In 1773 God was still in His Heaven, the maker and shaker
of all things. So, in 1798, when Jenner wrote the account
of his work leading to the vaccination against smallpox, he
began with the pietistical statement, "The deviation of man
from the state in which he was originally placed by nature
seems to have proved to him a prolific source of disease.
From the love of luxury and his fondness for amusement
he has familiarised himself with a great number of animals,
which may not have been intended for his associates." Not
for one hundred years would Pasteur replace this sybaritic
notion of disease with pathogenic bacteria.

These attributes of Jenner—physician, countryman,
naturalist, and moralist—led him to speculate on smallpox,
the most savage and disfiguring disease of eighteenth-century England. In every village, town, and city of Europe
those with stigmata of the diseases's aftermath were commonly seen. For every living pockmarked body, the grave
held another who did not survive the infection.

Jenner noted a disease affecting the hooves of horses,
which farriers called "the grease." The grease[1] was an
inflammatory condition with an exudation of purulent matter which Jenner (wrongly) believed to be infectious to cows.
Once the grease attacked the cow Jenner thought the con-

1. The "grease" is not a familiar clinical entity to today's veterinarians.
My vet friends think that it was a bacterial infection of the hooves.

tagion underwent a modification in that animal to produce cowpox. Since cowpox produces pustules of the cow's udder, Jenner was struck by the similarity of those symptoms to those of smallpox. Jenner began by betting on the wrong horse, but once he switched to the cow he got on the right epidemiological track. Jenner knew that dairymaids and others who milked poxy cows often came down with the cowpox-like, self-limiting sickness characterized by fever and small pustules of the hands that soon healed. He next made an Olympian observational leap in discerning that those who had had cowpox never become infected with smallpox: "Morbid matter of various kinds, when absorbed into the system, may produce effects in some degrees similar; but what renders the cowpox virus[2] so extremely singular is that the person who has been thus affected is forever after secure from the infection of smallpox."

Jenner then began to put his theory to the test of human experimentation. What he did would be forbidden today, but in eighteenth-century England there were no committees on human experimentation and few rules. Jenner obtained pauper children from the workhouse or from peasant families and inoculated them with pus from the cowpox pustules followed sometime later with an inoculating challenge of material taken from the pustules of someone stricken with smallpox.[3]

2. Jenner's use of the term "virus" was both amorphous and prescient since the microbial nature of infectious diseases was not known at that time. The first virus discovered was one of plants—the tobacco mosaic virus—in 1892 by Iwanowski in Russia. The yellow fever virus, discovered in 1900 by the U.S. Army Commission led by Major Walter Reed, was the first human viral disease to be identified.

3. I wrote this chapter during a period of residence at the Rockefeller Foundation's Study Center, the Villa Seberlloni in Bellagio, Italy, where I had the good fortune to have as a companion scholar-in-residence the Reverend Professor Maurice Wiles of Oxford University who has both

In May of 1796 he selected an eight-year-old boy and inoculated him with "matter taken from the sore hand of a dairymaid." The next day the boy became ill—fever, headache, loss of appetite—but the following day he was completely well again. Several months later Jenner inoculated the child with "matter" taken from a smallpox pustule. The child was protected; no disease occurred. The experiment was a success and the human species (and their domestic animals) began to secure the protection of immunization.

Jenner unaccountably discontinued these human experiments for two years until in March 1778 he inoculated a five year old with cowpox, although this child was "rendered unfit for inoculation (with smallpox) from having felt the effects of a contagious fever in a workhouse." A month later he inoculated three girls, ages five, six, and seven, and two infant boys, eleven and twelve months old. However, it was Jenner's nonphysician nephew, a Mr. Henry Jenner, who was left to complete the trial by challenging the children with smallpox pus to determine if they were protected. To make sure that he had "hot" pus for the challenge, Henry Jenner inoculated a "patient" who had not been vaccinated with cowpox. Subsequently he was happy to report to his uncle that this "produced smallpox in the

an encyclopedic knowledge of the ethics and beliefs of Jenner's time and a very wicked forehand slice. I discussed with him my problem in trying to reconcile Jenner's religious convictions and the nobleness of his scientific aims with his exploitive use of children as experimental subjects. Professor Wiles explained that the Protestant God of eighteenth-century England was considered to care only for the upper and middle social classes. The poor were beyond His protection because they had committed the sin of being born poor; they were children of a lesser breed. And so, in all probability Jenner felt no ethical compunction in using these pauper children as guinea pigs. In the ethical-religious climate of the day, they were at least serving a better purpose than that for which they were born.

regular manner." We can only wonder what the afflicted "patient" thought of this experiment.

The medical profession was at first reluctant to accept Jenner's discovery, but by 1802 most opposition had diminished and vaccination became commonplace. In 1807 the government of Bavaria passed a law making vaccination compulsory and by the early twentieth century smallpox was, essentially, cornered in the tropical regions. Then in the 1970s a masterful campaign was undertaken in which the strategy was to identify and vaccinate all the smallpox contacts in all parts of the endemic tropics. This campaign, ten years after its inception, exterminated the virus.

When the calendar turned its page to the nineteenth century, humankind possessed the crucial element of knowledge, prised from human experimentation, that an experience with a deliberately induced mild form of infection could produce a very solid protection—an immunity—against a related pathogenic infection. That the cowpox-smallpox was the first of such immunizing relationships discovered proved fortuitous. Obviously, many infectious experiences, such as influenza or the common cold, are only very narrowly protective and do not lead to the relatively broad, strong immunity of vaccination against the smallpox virus by its cowpox relative.

Even so, as important and as immensely practical as Jenner's discovery was, it was a discovery made in intellectual isolation. The scientific knowledge of the microbial causation of disease was not then available to allow its extension to other immunizations. And so, vaccination (or more accurately, artificial immunization) remained in limbo for another hundred years until Pasteur revealed the pathogenic potential of bacteria.

*Chapter 2*

# Mr. Pasteur's
# Chicken Shot Becomes a
# Barrage

THIS IS a book about immunology, but the evolution of that science is intertwined with that of bacteriology. The two must be considered together. Louis Pasteur, the chemist of Dijon, is our grand model. Not only was Pasteur the first to prove that certain bacteria are pathogenic, he was also the first to demonstrate that when these bacteria are modified they can, through immunization, induce protection against themselves. Like many other "monumental" discoveries of biomedical science, Pasteur arrived at these findings in a circuitous, serendipitous way. The modern scientific establishment, supplicating and scrambling for funds and recognition, would have us believe in the powerful and orderly logic by which "breakthroughs" are made. The truth is that this is no truer today than it was in Pasteur's day. More often than not the "big discovery" is made by chance; the crucial phenomenon is observed while looking for something else, perhaps completely unrelated. Logic and explanations come later. The true genius of those who make the great discoveries from chance observations is that they *recognize* significance and implication. Pasteur said it all when he said that "chance favors the prepared mind."

This serendipity principle surely applies to bacteriology, the origins of which stem not from the contemplation of the nature of human disease but from an inquiry on the morbid causes of a wine gone bad. Pasteur was, after all, not only a chemist but also a patriotic Frenchman. He knew what was important to the nation—a good bottle of wine and an understanding as to how the grape is transformed into a *grand cru*.

Wine had, of course, been made for at least two thousand years before Pasteur undertook his investigations, but the ancients thought that their amphora of "plonk" came from a kind of intrinsic, spontaneous generation taking place within the grape juice. Pasteur theorized wine to be a product of a chemical process, the conversion of sugar into alcohol (fermentation), and he discovered the yeast organism to be the agent for this process. He isolated the yeast and demonstrated that it can perform the miracle of transforming sterile sugar water into alcohol. What is more, he found that this can take place in the near total absence of oxygen (anaerobic conditions).

From his discovery that yeast ferments sugar, Pasteur conjured a world of microorganisms whose activities are manifest not only for useful purposes—as in grapes-to-wine—but also in harmful ways—as a "wild yeast" that would make a fermentation go sour. In his search for bad *microbes* (a term coined not by Pasteur but by one of his colleagues, a Monsieur Sedillot), his attention was drawn to the "sicknesses" of wine and beer (he believed that despite the outcome of Franco-Prussian War a Frenchman should make better beer than a German—an ambition which remains unrealized), and to a disease, pébrine, which was killing silkworms and causing serious economic loss to the French silk industry. In each case—for the wine gone sour, the beer turned bitter, and the dying silkworms—he found a specific causative microorganism. Diseases of domestic animals next came under his experimental scrutiny and he discovered that bacteria are the causative agents of anthrax of sheep and of fowl cholera. Thus, he proved that microbes endanger the health not only of beer, wine, and silkworms, but also of vertebrate animals. Man and his diseases were only one experimental step away. In the late 1870s, Pasteur went searching for—and found—bacteria in patients with septicemia and osteomyelitis (infections of the blood and bone, respectively).

In proving the bacterial etiology (cause) of these conditions, Pasteur employed an experimental method in which he isolated and grew the bacteria of these diseases in a sterile culture medium which was usually akin to a consommé of chicken or beef. The bacteria were isolated by diluting matter taken from a diseased animal or human and inoculated into the culture broth. When the broth was teeming with microbes he then, in the case of animal diseases, injected some of the broth into a "clean" animal to determine whether or not the disease would be produced. For example, in isolating the anthrax bacillus (a bacillus is a rod-shaped bacterium), *B. anthracis,* he proportionally diluted the material from the diseased sheep "in a volume of (culture) fluid equal to the total volume of the earth." The bacilli flourished in the culture medium and, when a small amount of the culture fluid—now containing numerous, rapidly dividing microbes—was inoculated into a sheep, anthrax resulted. But from one such experiment, an experiment that "went wrong," mankind was propelled along the road to protective immunization.

By 1887, Pasteur was established in his own laboratory in Paris (now the renowned Pasteur Institute) working on the cause of fowl cholera, a killing diarrheic disease of chickens. From stricken chickens he isolated in culture a bacillus now known as *Pasturella antiseptica*. After a few days, the cultures became infectious and produced the typical disease when inoculated into experimental fowl. However, in one experiment Pasteur let his cultures incubate longer than usual before transferring the microbes into fresh medium. We don't know the reason for his delay although every married scientist can imagine an encounter in which an exasperated Mrs. Pasteur might say, "What, Louis, you are going to the laboratory today? This is the weekend you promised to clean out the closets." Whatever the predisposing circumstances, when Pasteur injected the now relatively aged culture of microbes into chickens nothing happened. The animals didn't develop fowl cholera. At the time, Pasteur thought nothing of this except perhaps the frustration that all scientists experience from time to time when a routine procedure fails for no apparent reason. Pasteur, however—as frugal as any budget-conscious researcher today—didn't discard these "failed" chickens and a few weeks later when he had fresh cultures of "strong" fowl cholera bacilli he reinoculated these same chickens. But the birds *still* didn't become infected—they were *resistant* to a challenge of virulent organisms. A lesser mind would have discarded the experiment as hopelessly botched (and eaten the chickens) but Pasteur incisively realized that by "aging" the microbes in culture they had been made, somehow, less virulent—attenuated. Having lost their ability to cause disease they induced an immunity.

This established a basic principle of immunization with vaccines: a microbial pathogen modified or manipulated in a way that renders it harmless induces a protective immunity in otherwise susceptible animals or humans. Indeed, for this and other findings, immunology is as much beholden to the chicken as is Colonel Sanders.

Pasteur's discoveries on the microbial causation of certain diseases had a profound effect on the way physicians viewed illness. Prior to Pasteur, physicians classified illness according to symptoms. After Pasteur, diagnosis of causation (etiology) became the primary concept for the treatment and prevention of disease. Moreover, unlike Jenner's work on smallpox a hundred years before, Pasteur's findings did not abort in intellectual isolation, but ushered in the age of microbiology and immunology, disciplines which continue to bubble and ferment like the yeast which gave them birth.

# Chapter 3

# The Thorn in the Starfish: Élie Metchnikoff and the Beginnings of Immunology

A FRENCHMAN'S thoughts on the nature of wine gave birth to bacteriology, but it was a Russian's contemplation of starfish digestion that gave first life to immunology.

When Pasteur vaccinated his chickens with attenuated bacterial cultures and protected them from fowl cholera, neither he nor anyone else of that time understood the immunological mechanisms involved. In fact, Pasteur was on the wrong theoretical foot in postulating that protection was due to a "nutritive exhaustion"; that is, he believed the attenuated bacteria consumed and depleted an essential nutriment present in the chicken's body which the virulent bacteria needed if they were to survive and multiply.[1] Those first clues to immunity's secrets were to be detected by Élie Metchnikoff, a Russian scientist who was supported and befriended by Pasteur. It was Metchnikoff who revealed that the body possessed an army of specialized cells whose

1. Pasteur wasn't *entirely* wrong. Certain conditions, such as low iron levels in the blood, prevent microbes from multiplying. This "nutritional immunity" is discussed in Chapter 7.

unique function is to scavenge, ingest, and destroy foreign particles such as invading bacteria. That the body could defend itself and that a specialized system of cells existed to do this was a daring and revolutionary proposal at that time. Only someone as brilliant, contentious, and moodily eccentric as Élie Metchnikoff could have defended his beloved scavenger cells against the medical disbelievers of the late nineteenth century.

In the cartoon strip "The Wizard of Id," Sir Rodney asks the King "Why are athletes worshipped and scientists go unnoticed?" The King answers, "Would you buy a ticket to see a scientist?" "No" says Rodney. "There you are," says the King, and so it is today. But that was not quite the case during my adolescent years of the late 1930s and early 1940s. Scientists then held a colorful affection in the popular mind. While not esteemed as highly as athletes—there wasn't a Louis Pasteur card that could be traded for a Louis Gehrig card—scientists were hailed on screen and in print. Paul Muni as Louis Pasteur is indelibly fused in my memory. Sinclair Lewis's Martin Arrowsmith must be one of the noblest characters in fiction. Biographers praised the lives of scientists. De Kruif's *Microbe Hunters* turned a generation of nascent researchers to microbiology. From the age of thirteen, when I first read *Microbe Hunters*, my greatest affection has continued to be for that quirky genius, Élie Metchnikoff. Never mind that even an admiring biographer called his subject a "gold mine for a psychoanalytically inclined biographer."[2] I like Metchnikoff's style; so let me exercise the privilege of old professors to digress, and tell you something of his life.

2. Gert H. Brieger's introduction to Metchnikoff's *Immunity in Infective Disease*, 1905, reprint (New York: Johnson Reprint Corporation, 1968).

Élie Metchnikoff was born in 1845 in the land of Pan-askova, the steppe of Little Russia where the country is "neither beautiful nor rich: steppes, hillocks covered with low grasses and wild wormwood; a poor village, meagre vegetation, no river: the whole impression is a melancholy one. But what boundless space!"[3] His father was a retired military officer, a landowner, a Christian. His mother, the daughter of the writer Leo Nevahovitch, was Jewish—although she couldn't have been what we now consider the stereotypic Jewish mother because she discouraged Metch-nikoff from becoming a physician. She felt he was too "sen-sitive" for that profession.

In 1862, the seventeen-year-old Metchnikoff decided to become a zoologist. He travelled to the University of Wurzburg in Germany to begin a series of confused mis-adventures that were to plague his entire life. Metchnikoff thought the term began in September only to find the Uni-versity deserted. The term began in October. Lonely and discouraged he fled back to Panaskova and, later in the year, entered the University of Kharkov where he blazed through and graduated after two years of study. Germany still beckoned however as the center of science and in 1864 he went to the University of Giessen with the intention of doing graduate study in parasitology under the famed Rudolf Leuckart, a man who has been called the Father of Exper-imental Parasitology. At Giessen, Metchnikoff undertook a study on the life cycle of *Ascaris nigrovenosa*, a round-worm (nematode) of frogs, and soon after made a remark-able discovery: *A. nigrovenosa* undergoes an alteration of generations. It first reproduces by sexual means and then

3. Olga Metchnikoff, *The Life of Elie Metchnikoff*, (Boston: Houghton Mifflin, 1921).

by asexual process, parthenogenesis (a kind of "virgin birth" in which the female doesn't require male sperm to produce a fertile egg).

This was just too good a discovery for a mere graduate student, and what happened next in the Metchnikoff-Leuckart relationship is sure to ring a sympathetic note for doctoral students everywhere who have to get a piece of their professor's action in order to carry out their dissertation research. Leuckart, according to Metchnikoff, first encouraged him to work out the details, then took the information and published it under his own name with only a passing reference in the paper to Metchnikoff. This first disappointment and acrimonious conflict with a High Priest of Research (alas) turned Metchnikoff away from parasitology. He left Giessen, as his wife Olga notes in her biography, "without taking leave of Leuckart."

The Russian government came to his assistance and awarded him a fellowship to enable him to work at the marine biological laboratory in Naples. There he fell in with another young Russian biologist, Kovalevsky, whose passion for zoology was equal to Metchnikoff's. Together they traced the development of the sponge from its postfertilization celluar origin to the separation and transformation of those cells into the specialized tissues of digestive tract and nervous system. Later, he was to return to, and build upon, those studies in formulating his concepts of the cellular organization of the immune system.

In 1867, Metchnikoff, now only twenty-two and a rising zoological star, obtained a teaching appointment at the University of Odessa (where he again arrived too early) and almost immediately had a fight with a senior professor over which of them should attend a scientific meeting. He left Odessa within the year to become professor of zoology at

Petersburg, but almost immediately after assuming that appointment he returned to Naples and the sponges. Again he collaborated with Kovalevsky but this time the great and good friends had a falling out over the way a sponge's nervous system develops (Kovalevsky's view eventually proved to be the correct one). Metchnikoff returned to Petersburg and came to despise his life there—the primitive laboratory facilities, the loneliness of his single life, his impecunious economic circumstances.

During the arctic Petersburg winter he became ill and was nursed to health by Ludmilla Fedorovitch, a daughter of a friend. Not exactly in love, he was fond of Ludmilla, and grateful. They became engaged, although to his beloved mother Metchnikoff gloomily predicted that "a rosy, boundless beatitude forms no part of my conception of the distant future." The idea of parenthood didn't fit into his plans, either, as he candidly wrote to Mama : "I intend to have no children—it is an embryologist who is speaking." Why an embryologist would be soured on the bread and butter of his profession is hard to understand, and certainly not a common attitude amongst those specialists: within my limited circle of acquaintances I have yet to meet a celibate embryologist. But Metchnikoff's forebodings were in fact tragically well founded. Before they were married Ludmilla contracted tuberculosis and grew so sick that she had to be carried to the church for the wedding ceremony.

The year was 1869 and Metchnikoff was twenty-five years old. He hated his Petersburg job; his wife was desperately ill, and he became paranoiacally distrustful of his colleagues. So once again he packed it in, and having obtained a modest research fellowship, left Petersburg for Spezzia, Italy, where he returned to his research on the embryology of the starfish. A year later the Metchnikoffs went home to

Russia; he to take up a teaching post in Odessa, Ludmilla to take an advised course of fermented mare's milk, *koumiss*, which was believed to cure tuberculosis. Koumiss failed to halt the progression of Ludmilla's disease, but they heard of miraculous cures for tuberculosis on the island of Maderia, to which they travelled from Odessa—a nightmare of a journey, considering the transportation of the time and Ludmilla's frail state of health.

Madeira, alas, proved no more therapeutic than mare's milk. Ludmilla's health continued to deteriorate, and on the 20th of April 1873, she died. Metchnikoff, overwhelmed by deep despair, went to Geneva, where his brother lived, and while there attempted suicide by taking an overdose of morphia. He miscalculated the lethal dose and took an amount not quite enough to do him in. As he emerged from the morphine coma he looked out his bedroom window and saw a cloud of mayflies flying, surging, during their brief moment of life, around a lantern. The curiosity of the biologist triumphed over his deep, semicomatose depression and Metchnikoff began to ponder on how the Darwinian laws of natural selection could apply to these insects. Olga writes: "His thoughts turned to science; he was saved; the link with life was re-established."

Two years later (1875) we find Metchnikoff back at the University of Odessa and remarried—this time to a young woman, Olga, who is a teenager, to Metchnikoff's thirty-one. Olga, despite her youth, was of a sterner and firmer constitution than the ill-fated Ludmilla and she was to be Metchnikoff's help, comfort, and collaborator until his death in 1916. However, even a new marriage didn't make a new Metchnikoff. In Odessa, he engaged in political fights— almost always on the losing side—in a university seething

with conflict between political conservatives and revolu-
tionaries.

Olga was stricken with typhoid and he nursed her back
to health. He was overworked; his eyesight was failing; he
imagined he had heart disease; he couldn't sleep. He was,
in 1881, an extremely depressed man and once again
attempted suicide. This time he chose a curious instrument
of death. He didn't want to make the suicide too obvious,
in order to spare his family's feelings, and being the constant scientist he wanted to make an "experiment" of his
death—an adventure in furthering knowledge. He inoculated himself with the blood of a person suffering from
relapsing fever[4] but he was no better a microbiologist in
estimating the lethality of the infection than he had been a
pharmacologist twelve years earlier in judging the mortal
dose of morphia. As Metchnikoff quickly discovered, the
microbe of relapsing fever *could* be transmitted by blood
passage. He was also to discover that this very nasty disease
brings a series of episodes of intense muscle pain, prolonged fever, nausea, jaundice, and delirium to its victims.
But it is not usually fatal—only 2 to 8 percent die of the
infection and most patients make a natural recovery, as
Metchnikoff did. (Now it can be successfully treated with
antibiotics.)

During his convalescence his mood rebounded. Olga
came into a modest inheritance that allowed Metchnikoff
to resign from the University of Odessa and its unhappy,

4. The causative organism of relapsing rever, *Borrelia recurrentis*, is a
microbe related to the spirochete of syphilis. It was first described by
Obermeier in 1868. Under natural conditions it is transmitted from person to person by a louse or a tick. From early times, great epidemics of
relapsing fever, often accompanied by louse-born typhus, swept through
Europe.

Byzantine political conflicts. In 1882, the reconstituted Metchnikoffs settled in Messina, where he was to begin his great work on phagocytosis—the research that was to occupy and buoyantly sustain him for the remainder of his life.

At the Messina marine biology laboratory, work was resumed on the embryology of sea anemones (coelenterates) and starfish (echinoderms). Metchnikoff paid special attention to the cellular origins of the digestive tract. Within certain cells lining the intestine of these primitive animals he noticed minute morsels. These cells had actively ingested the microscopic organic minutiae of the sea, which is their source of food. Metchnikoff carried out an experiment to observe this activity by introducing grains of carmine dye into the mouth-like opening of a living sea anemone. The digestive cells were seen to form amoeba-like extrusions, which captured the foreign particles and brought them within the cell.[5] Metchnikoff, the biologist who thought in terms of natural laws governing all living animals, seized upon the idea that ingestion by specialized cells (he was later to call them *phagocytes*) was the means by which both low and high creatures, including man, defended themselves against foreign bodies—even hostile foreign bodies such as dis-

5. When he hypothesized on the evolutionary geneology of the immune system, of which he considered the phagocytic cell to be the cornerstone, it seems to me that Metchnikoff did not descend far enough down the "tree." The great evolutionary step that was to lead, eventually, to the mammals, occurred when the earth was very young and there appeared that single-celled protozoan—the amoeba. The amoeba was presumably the first organism that did not passively absorb nutriments from the surrounding environmental "soup" or obtain energy, plant-fashion, from sunlight. The amoeba actively captured food. This seems a simple act but, in fact, it is immeasurably complex because to capture the food the amoeba would have to recognize the food: to discern it as being different—non-self. Its outer membrane would have to possess a sensory function, probably in the form of chemical receptors. In a way, this first discrimination between self and non-self to obtain food, was the beginning of consciousness—the beginning of personality.

ease-causing microbes. When this grand concept burst upon him (Metchnikoff's account):

> I was resting from the shock of the events which provoked my resignation from the University and indulging enthusiastically in researches in the splendid setting of the Straits of Messina.
>
> One day when the whole family had gone to a circus to see some extraordinary performing apes, I remained alone with my microscope, observing the life in the mobile cells of a transparent star-fish larva, when a new thought suddenly flashed across my brain. It struck me that similar cells might serve in the defence of the organism against intruders. Feeling that there was in this something of surpassing interest, I felt so excited that I began striding up and down the room and even went to the seashore to collect my thoughts.
>
> I said to myself that, if my supposition were true, a splinter introduced into the body of a star-fish larva, devoid of blood-vessels or of a nervous system, should soon be surrounded by mobile cells as is to be observed in a man who runs a splinter into his finger. This was no sooner said than done.
>
> There was a small garden in our dwelling, in which we had a few days previously organized a "Christmas tree" for the children on a little tangerine tree: I fetched from it a few rose thorns and introduced them at once under the skin of some beautiful star-fish larvae as transparent as water.
>
> I was too excited to sleep that night in the expectation of the results of my experiment, and very early the next morning I ascertained that it had fully succeeded.
>
> That experiment formed the basis of the phagocyte theory, to the development of which I devoted the next twenty-five years of my life.

From that moment on, Metchnikoff began to think more like a medical researcher than the biologist-naturalist of his former years. His first extension of the phagocyte theory to humans was to try to explain the cells abundant in pus. In 1883, when Metchnikoff met the phagocyte, it was known from (1) Pasteur's work that boils were caused by certain pathogenic bacteria which invade a localized area of the skin and, from (2) the work of others that the viscous fluid within the boil (pus) contained not only bacteria but also large numbers of white blood cells (leukocytes).[6] Several years earlier, the German pathologists Cohnheim and Virchow had shown that the leukocytes which normally circulate in the blood could insinuate themselves through the walls of the blood vessels to accumulate at an infected, inflamed site—such as a boil. Others, including the doyen bacteriologist Robert Koch, had noted the presence of bacteria within some leukocytes but did not associate this as evidence of a defense mechanism. In fact, Koch believed that these leukocytes were the vehicle which spread the infection to other parts of the body.[7]

Metchnikoff was the first to recognize the curative attributes of phagocytic cells.[8] In 1887, now forty-seven, he

6. Blood, "the nimble spirit in the arteries," as Shakespeare described it, is composed of formed elements—the red blood cells (erythrocytes), white blood cells (leukocytes), and platelets—suspended in a chemically complex fluid medium, the plasma (*serum* when the clotting factor has been removed). Erythrocytes are the hemoglobin-containing cells that transport the oxygen necessary for the respiration of the body's tissues. Leukocytes are a diverse family of nucleated cells that have many immunological functions including phagocytosis (Chapters 6 and 7). Platelets are small, unnucleated cells involved in blood clot formation. A constituent of plasma is immunoglobulin(s) which is the antibody of the immune reaction (Chapters 4 and 5).

7. Koch wasn't entirely mistaken. Certain microbes such as the protozoan *Leishmania*, the cause of kala-azar, have made the remarkable adaptation to live, in an obligate relationship, entirely within the phagocyte. Other pathogens such as the bacterium causing brucellosis (undulant fever) can survive and multiply within the phagocyte.

8. Collectively, the cells that ingest particles have retained Metchnikoff's original designation of *phagocytes*. However, phagocytes are a family of very different cells whose names have undergone changes over the years. Metchnikoff recognized a phagocytic cell with a lobed nucleus which he termed *microphage* and a cell with a round nucleus to which he gave the name *macrophage*. In today's phagocyte libretto, the microphage has become the *polymorphonuclear leucocyte (PMN)*. *Macrophage* is a term now reserved for round-nucleated phagocytic cells that are fixed to tissues (like a sponge to a rock), chiefly to blood vessel linings

travelled to Paris to meet Pasteur. The Pasteur Institute was then under construction and Metchnikoff requested laboratory space to continue his work on the phagocyte— no pay, just laboratory facilities. Pasteur agreed and a year later the Metchnikoffs settled in the outskirts of Paris, where they were to remain for the rest of their lives.

At the Pasteur Institute, Metchnikoff and his French colleagues demonstrated that the phagocytes are active in a great variety of bacterial infections. In the course of this research they became convinced that they had discovered the single supreme mechanism of immunity. But during this time other research had been carried out, mainly in Germany, that pointed to another arm of the immune system: a noncellular, soluble factor in the blood serum.

Metchnikoff, now totally enamored with his phago-cytes, adamantly refused to accept the growing evidence for the serum immune factor and for the next few years there raged the Franco-German War of Immunity. Of course both contestants were right. It is now known that there is an intimate, crucial interdependence between the cellular and serum (humoral) arms of the immune system. In fact, the phagocytes are now known to have immunological functions that Metchnikoff never dreamed of. The Father of the Phagocyte would be proud of them if he were alive today.

of spleen and liver. The round-nucleated phagocytes that circulate in the blood and wander to the tissues when needed are called *monocytes* or *monocyte macrophages*. More of these cells in later chapters.

# Chapter 4

# The Humors of
# Immunity

VERY FEW physicians in the Western world
will ever see a case of diphtheria. Sixty years ago it was
quite different. Diphtheria, a common disease and a great
child killer, brought thousands to a cruel death from suffo-
cation as the dirty white membranes induced by the multiplying bacteria occluded the airway passages of the lungs
and throat. From the 1930s onward, effective immunization and various new forms of therapy drastically reduced
the incidence of the disease, although, in parts of the Third
World where immunizations and drugs are a luxury, death
by diphtheria is still commonplace.

In the years following Pasteur's proofs of the germ theory of disease, the science of bacteriology progressed with
remarkable rapidity. The new science was quickly taken up
(or "appropriated," if you were French) by the Germans
and new findings bounced back and forth from France to
Germany to France. In 1883, only three years after Pasteur
startled the medical profession by announcing that boils were
caused by bacteria, a German scientist by the name of Klebs
described a club-shaped bacterium (a bacillus now called
*Corynebacterium diphtheriae*) in the material obtained from
throat swabs of patients suffering from diphtheria. A year
later, another German bacteriologist, Löffler, proved it to

be the causative organism of the disease and worked out a method for growing the bacteria in culture medium.

Now over to France where, in 1888, two scientists at the Pasteur Institute, Roux and Yersin, performed an experiment to determine whether they could produce typical diphtheria in a rabbit by inoculating the animal with culture medium containing living bacilli. To their amazement the rabbit didn't become *progressively* ill, as is typical of diphtheria. It died almost *immediately* following the injection. A powerful substance in the culture fluid, a toxin more potent than a viper's venom, had been secreted by the bacillus. It was this toxin that brought a halt to the rabbit heart's vital rhythmic beat (an effect that also occurs in some human patients with diphtheria). Several months later, a similarly powerful toxin was discovered in the culture fluid in which the tetanus bacillus had been grown.

Events now moved rapidly. In the closing weeks of 1890 the German, Emil von Behring, and his Japanese partner, Shibasaburo Kitasato, working in Robert Koch's[1] Institut für Infektionskrankheiten (infectious diseases) in Berlin announced their discovery of a completely new dimension to the immune system. In their paper, published in the December 3, 1890, issue of the *Berliner klinische Wochenschrift,* they described experiments in which they had injected rabbits with minute, nonlethal amounts of tetanus toxin derived from bacterial cultures. Several weeks later they obtained serum from these rabbits and inoculated it into mice shortly after the mice had been given the full, lethal dose of toxin. The mice not only survived but also

1. Robert Koch (1843–1910) is generally acknowledged as the founder of modern bacteriology. He established the main principles of specific culture methods and systematic bacteriology. He also discovered the causative bacteria of tuberculosis and cholera.

exhibited no sign whatsoever of the toxin's poisonous effect. A week later, von Behring published another paper describing the same experiment and the same results with the diphtheria bacillus toxin. Clearly, some substance in serum of injected (immunized) rabbits neutralized bacterial toxin. Behring named this serum element *antitoxin*.

This was great science, but was it good medicine? Children not mice died of diphtheria. Would the antitoxin halt and cure the disease? There was a preciously small stock of antitoxin and in Berlin, on Christmas Eve of 1891, it was given to a child who lay stricken with diphtheria, her life ebbing away in agonizing gasps. The prospect for survival had seemed hopeless. The physician, a Doctor Giessler, requested, and obtained, a vial of the antitoxin and in a moment of high drama slowly infused the serum into the dying child's vein. By morning the fever had broken, the membranes had receded, and breathing became less labored. Life had been restored by the antitoxin. In the ensuing years the lives of thousands suffering from diphtheria were saved by the miracle of antitoxic serum.[2] In those later years the antitoxin(s) were produced in "bulk" by immunizing horses.

The great antitoxin hunt now commenced, and a giant new intellect, Paul Ehrlich, stepped on to the immunological stage to put a tidy Germanic order to the confusion that

2. Similar to many other "breakthroughs" of medical science, antitoxin therapy was initially seen as the universal cure for all bacteria-caused diseases. But most bacteria do not produce toxins and except for diphtheria and tetanus, antitoxin proved no more a therapeutic philosopher's stone than has modern day antibiotics. With the advent of specific immunization and chemotherapy with the sulfa drugs in the 1930s, antitoxic therapy for diphtheria and tetanus became a rarely used measure. This type of "passive immune therapy" is now mainly reserved to the giving of antivenins (antitoxins to venoms) in the treatment of snakebites.

surrounded the nature and application of antitoxins. When Ehrlich began his researches, not long after the first human use, antitoxins were given in a rather trial and error fashion. It was uncertain how much to inject into the patient because the dose was not standardized and the potency of the antitoxic serum varied from preparation to preparation.

Ehrlich was like a Silesian mirror image of the French Pasteur. Pasteur was a chemist who thought like a physician while Ehrlich was a physician who thought like a chemist. It was the "chemical" side of their natures that led them to view biological phenomena in terms of chemical reactions—how the elements come together to form bonded molecular complexes; the quantitative, measurable, ways in which those reactions occurred. Ehrlich attacked the toxins like a chemist. He put one (toxin) and one (antitoxin) together and saw that they combined in quantitative proportions: so much antitoxin neutralized just so much of a toxin. These studies were not only of great theoretical interest but they also led to the technology that enabled antitoxins and, eventually, other therapeutic biologic substances (such as insulin and hormones) to be standardized. Without that standardization they could not be used for the treatment of humans except on an experimental basis.

So far, all the known toxins had been bacterial products and there was a vague notion that they were all of a kind. Ehrlich pointed out, however, that toxic substances might flow from other sources. One of these was ricin, a powerfully lethal substance in the bean of the castor plant. Another plant toxin was abrin, derived from the seed of the rosary pea. What Ehrlich did next established a fundamental principle of immunity and is crucial to our understanding of how immune reactions operate. In these experiments Ehrlich first made, in rabbits, an antitoxin against ricin. This antitoxin protected mice from the lethal effects of that toxin, as expected. Next, Ehrlich injected mice with *abrin* and tried to protect them with an inoculation of the *ricin* antitoxin. Nothing happened. The mice died. Vice versa, when he made an antitoxin to abrin it would not protect (neutralize) ricin. Thus, Ehrlich showed that antitoxin is *specific:* it only works against the toxin which promoted its formation. Ehrlich now began to formulate his theory that the toxin and antitoxin possessed, by virtue of their respective chemical compositions, a unique structural configuration that allowed them to fit together as a key would to a lock. Ricin antitoxin could not save the mice from abrin because the "tumblers" of that antitoxin were "set" in a different pattern than the "key" of abrin. Similarly a diphtheria antitoxin would not help a patient stricken with tetanus. As we shall see repeatedly during the course of this book, specificity is the *modus operandi* of the great majority of immune reactions.[3]

During the decade that followed Behring's and Ehrlich's discoveries, there was a novalike explosion of research on antitoxins. The work of scientists in France, Germany, England, and the United States revealed that this serum factor, now renamed *antibody,* could be raised not only

3. Meanwhile, in the midst of all this research Ehrlich was fathering the science of chemopharmacology (therapy by chemically-synthesized drugs). Actually, immunology and chemotherapy were not so disparate in Ehrlich's point of view. Both antitoxin (antibody) and drugs combined with their targets, toxins and microbes, because of specific chemical lock-and-key fittings. Curiously, the organic dye industry which was beginning to flourish in late nineteenth-century Germany was the springboard to this concept. Ehrlich noted that certain dyes would stain—combine with—only certain microbes. This led Ehrlich to the idea that these dyes could act as "magic bullets"—guided missiles, really—to act as specific curative agents. Ehrlich's successful search for the "magic bullet" to cure syphilis came from this idea. That bullet, an organic arsenical, salvarsan, was based on a variation of a dye's formula.

against bacterial and plant toxins but also developed in response to whole bacteria and other pathogens. In the test tube, the reaction of antibody and pathogen could actually be seen when the two were mixed together. The organisms clumped together, a precipitate was formed with the toxin or soluble extract of the pathogen, or the offending pathogen was killed and dissolved (lysed).[4] In the latter event, a Belgian scientist, Jules Bordet, showed in 1895 that for lysis to take place another, naturally occurring, element in the blood, *complement*, must participate with the antibody.

Finally, it was shown that antibodies arose not only against toxins and microbial pathogens but against any substance of sufficient size (molecular weight) and, in the chemical sense, structural complexity for the body to recognize as alien—as being different from self. Collectively, these substances, as different and diverse as red blood cell types, egg albumin, and pollen grains, were designated as *antigens*.

When the humors of immunity[5] were beginning to take

4. A subdiscipline of immunology, *serology*, is concerned with the diverse techniques for the "test-tube" demonstration and measurement of antibody reactions. Serologic techniques are applied not only for the diagnosis of present and past infections but also for other purposes such as blood typing. Indeed, without the serological methods to characterize donor and recipient blood types, blood transfusions would not be possible.

5. From Hippocrates until the mid–nineteenth century, it was believed that there were four different kinds of humors (fluids) in the human body—blood, phlegm, black bile, and yellow bile. Disease and personality disorders were thought to be caused by an imbalance of the humors (hence, bloodletting to redress the balance). Immunologists adopted the term "humoral" (of a body fluid) when they wanted to describe immunity brought about by the serum antibody. Such immunity is referred to a *humoral immunity*.

The sort of immunity Metchnikoff postulated was brought about by cellular elements, the phagocytes. This is referred to as *cellular immunity* or, in the expanded context of current immunological concepts, as *cell-mediated immunity*.

theoretical precedence over the phagocytes, Metchnikoff and his school of followers at the Pasteur Institute were denying it all. Antibody was merely a product of his beloved, but disintegrated, phagocytes—so Metchnikoff's (faulty) reasoning ran. But as we shall see in the succeeding chapters on modern concepts of the immune system, it was a false polemic. The cellurists and the humorists were both right. We know now that the cellular arm and the humoral arm of the immune system are intimately related and interact. In a way, the Nobel Prize committee of 1908 anticipated the marriage of the two schools by awarding the Prize for that year jointly to Metchnikoff and Ehrlich.

Thus, by 1910 the basic mechanisms of the immune system were known:

1. The body reacts and defends itself against substances it recognizes as foreign (antigens), that is, different from self.

2. It does this through two defensive arms: (A) specialized fixed and wandering cells (phagocytes) that devour foreign bodies such as invading bacteria; (B) the humoral arm, a substance (antibody) in the fluid (plasma / serum) portion of the blood that is elaborated in response to the foreigner (antigen) and will *specifically* combine with it and neutralize it. In that combination there is another, naturally occurring element in the plasma, *complement*, which participates in the killing (lysis) of the bacteria.

In the years following 1910, attention was focused on the humoral arm of the immune system. What was antibody? What was the source of its manufacture in the body? How did it act? It was to take another thirty years, however, before these questions were satisfactorily answered. The sophisticated tools the immunological trade required to probe these problems were not available in 1910.

During the intervening decades an allied science, bio-chemistry, was making logarithmic advances in research on the chemical composition of living creatures. Knowledge was being gained on how those chemicals functioned in life processes. The predominant building material of all living things, from ameobas to zebras, was found to be protein. Then, it was shown that all proteins are composed of twenty different amino acids strung end to end in an enormous molecular chain.[6] The character of the protein depends on the kinds and sequences of the amino acids in the chain. By the 1920s, it was realized that the major component of serum is protein and that antibody is a serum protein—although not all serum proteins are antibody.

In the late 1930s, the technical means became available to begin the characterization of antibody protein. The chemical composition of protein molecules is such that they carry an electrical charge. The magnitude of that charge differs for different proteins. A Swede, Arne Tiselius (later joined by a New Yorker, Elvin Kabat), exploited the electric potential of protein by passing a polarized current through serum in an apparatus devised for this purpose. Under these conditions the serum separated into four components which they labeled *gamma globulin, beta globulin, alpha globulin*, and a fast-moving fraction which was found to be albumin. When the serum from an immunized individual was separated by this process (electrophoresis), antibody was found to be mainly in the gamma globulin fraction.

---

6. The mode of assembly of the protein chain by living cells was revealed by the discovery and function of the genetic DNA. The DNA gene, contained within the cell's nucleus, is the coded tape issuing instructions as to which amino acids are to be spliced together in the proper sequence to construct that particular protein. The coded instruction is transmitted to the cell's RNA located in the cytoplasm outside the nucleus. It is the RNA which then actually assembles the protein.

Forty years later, and after at least forty elegant modifications of the original electrophoresis technique as well as entirely new methodologies, it has been shown that antibody is not a single class of globulin protein but a family of five classes which have been termed *immunoglobulin* (*Ig* in the immunologist's shorthand) *G*, *M*, *D*, *A*, and *E*. Each of these Ig's have their characteristic structure and function. In the next chapters, we shall learn something of those characteristics and the network of interacting specialized cells responsible for their formation as part of the body's immune response.

**II**

*The Owner's Manual on
the Immune System*

# Chapter 5

# The Immune System
# Turns On:
# Antigens and
# Antibodies

IF THIS were a textbook on immunology, I would begin this part of the book with a discourse on natural immunity. "Natural immunity" is a catchall for the barriers, inherent antimicrobial factors, and killer cells that "instinctively" recognize the aliens (antigens) and deal with them. Nothing is *provoked* into action in natural immunity. The opening historical chapters have, however, been leading our train of thought to *acquired immunity*, the specific induction by, and reaction to, foreign substances (the antigens). Since this is not a textbook but is designed to be read for pleasure, why break the rhythm? I'll stay with acquired immunity and come back later to immunity au naturel. Anyway, immunity is so circularly interdependent that there are several logical starting points. Primer fashion, let us begin with:

## A Is for ANTIGEN

Antigens switch on the immune system. Anything that turns you on, immunologically speaking, is an antigen. The immune system's specialized cells recognize the antigen as being foreign—different from self, not of the body corporate. These aliens may be life-threatening pathogens such as viruses, bacteria, and parasites. But in addition to the microbial pathogens there are an enormous diversity of other antigens. They can be cells, including blood cells, from other individuals and species. They can be drugs, including tobacco, and even cancer cells that form within our own body. And there are diseases, autoimmune diseases, where the immune system becomes "confused" and reacts against its own tissues as if they were foreign antigens.

Darwinian principles would explain an immune system that evolved to recognize and react against the pathogens that have been hammering at the human body for untold millennia. As we scaled the evolutionary tree, our parasites went along for the ride. A selectively defensive-protective immune system is compatible with the theory of natural selection; those individuals with traits that would limit a microbe's pathogenicity would be more fit to survive (and pass on those traits) than those individuals lacking the traits (genes) for effective immunity. But Darwin and his followers would be hard put to explain why animals (including us humans) respond to microbial and other antigens they have never, during the course of their evolution, met before. If it were merely a nonspecific, "blunderbuss" defense it would make a logical Darwinian fit. But our immune system is no blunderbuss. It is a system with the exquisitely specific virtuosity to recognize, molecule by molecule, virtually every antigen on Earth. The higher vertebrates have been endowed with an immune system to cope not only with the antigens we know but all the *future* antigens as well. Should a completely new microbial pathogen arise ten thousand years from now, the human immune system will be ready and waiting.

We perceive an immune reaction as being elicited against a bacterium, a flu virus, a pollen grain, a thirty-foot-long tapeworm. Operationally, that is not how it works. The entire microbe, for example, doesn't constitute an antigenic unit. The immune system reacts to the molecular components of the microbe. So in considering the nature of antigens we must think small, on the molecular level, smaller than any object that can be resolved by even the most powerful of electron microscopes. Antigens are of three chemical classes: proteins, complex carbohydrates (sugars), and fats. Fats are not very good as antigens but may induce an immune reaction when linked to proteins (lipoproteins). Similarly, sugars may also be bonded to proteins to form glycoproteins.

An immunological paradox for which there is still no satisfactory answer is that antigens must be big, in the molecular sense, to activate the immune system. A molecular weight[1] over 10,000 is required to initiate an immune response and, in general, the bigger the antigen molecule the more vigorous the immune reaction. The paradox is that the specific immune response(s) recognizes and reacts with only a very small "patch" of the antigen molecule. For example, a protein antigen molecule with a molecular weight

1. When the atoms of two or more elements combine to form a molecule, the compound formed will have a *molecular weight* which is the sum of its atomic parts. Thus water which is composed of two atoms of hydrogen (atomic weight hydrogen = 1) and one atom of oxygen (atomic weight oxygen = 16) has a molecular weight of 18 (decimals rounded off). Amino acids are composed of carbon, hydrogen, oxygen, and nitrogen atoms (a few amino acids also have sulfur atoms). For example, one amino acid, alanine, has three carbon atoms, seven hydrogen atoms, one nitrogen atom, and two oxygen atoms, which gives it a molecular weight of 89.

of 14,000 would consist of a chain of about 120 amino acids; but on that chain a patch, or patches, of only 6 to 20 amino acid sequences will act as the determinant of specificity. This knowledge stems from earlier studies in which immunochemists joined a simple, benzene-like organic compound to a "carrier" protein. By itself this chemical couldn't elicit antibody formation when inoculated into an experimental animal—its molecular weight was too low. However, antibody was produced to the conjoined compound and that antibody recognized, exclusively and specifically, the benzene-like chemical. Immunochemists now have elegant techniques which allow them to snip out pieces of the protein or polysaccharide (complex sugar) and "sew" these pieces onto another long-chain "carrier" molecule. They can then immunize an experimental animal with this hybrid antigen and show that the antibody formed is specific to the "patch" in the spliced antigen. These methods, as we shall describe in Chapter 13, are being used to identify the important "patches" to create new and potent vaccines.

In nature there are only twenty-two kinds of common amino acids. Each of these amino acids can be bonded to one another to form short chains (peptides) or long chains (proteins).[2] Biochemistry texts will illustrate these chains as configurations of C's (carbon atoms), H's (hydrogen atoms), O's (oxygen atoms) and N's (nitrogen atoms) with dash lines between them to represent the bonding relationships. The chemical formulas appear flat (two-dimensional) on the printed page. This is misleading and even confusing. As a student, I could never quite believe in the reality of chemistry's symbolic alphabet soup and I elected to pursue the

2. In the living organism, enzymes act as "welders" to connect the amino acids in "head-to-tail" fashion.

solidity that is biology. Alas, I was soon to realize that those palpable biological forms were made of chemicals and it was still necessary to comprehend chemistry. In fact, the amino acid chain is three-dimensional. It has form and substance. The shape—the physiognomy—of the six to twenty amino acid sequence in the peptide or protein chain that constitute the antigenic determinant "patch" (immunologists call the "patch" an *epitope*) is determined by the kind of constituent amino acids and their order of sequence. A substitution of a single amino acid with another kind of amino acid will change the shape of the epitope. The immune system is so exquisitely fine-tuned as to discriminate that single substitution and produce a uniquely specific antibody to the new configuration. Obviously, even given the limitation of twenty-two different amino acids in an epitope composed of only six amino acids allows for an enormous number of possible combinations—that is, an enormous number of possible antigens. One immunologist calculated that one billion different kinds of antigens (epitopes) are possible, but the mathematically minded reader with a home computer can verify this.

The diversity of amino acid combinations is essential not only for specificity but also for the very ability to provoke the immune reaction—to be antigenic. A string of amino acids or sugars is, in principle, like the synthetically bonded chain of molecules that make up Nylon, Orlon, and Teflon—a polymer. Life, in some respects, can be defined as The Big Polymer. There is, however, one essential difference between the polymers of nature and those of Du Pont. The polymers of our shirts and skirts are chemically uniform, one same molecule after another. For reasons that are still not clear, the immune system ignores this chemical monotony and does not respond to it. Probably, this uniformity doesn't give the stereoscopic shape needed for an antigen to be an antigen. It is for this reason that surgeons can implant Teflon valves in the heart and other plastic prosthetic devices without concern that an immune response, leading to rejection, will be mounted. Someone else's heart (or some other animal's heart) is a different antigenic matter. Each individual, except for identical twins and some highly inbred strains of experimental laboratory animals, carried a unique personal amino acid sequence code on the surface of each cell that would be recognized as antigenic (foreign) by another individual (who has a different personal epitope on his cells) after organ or tissue transplant. More of the donor-recipient, graft-versus-host problem later.

## A Is Also for ANTIBODY

Again, contrary to textbook exposition, I will continue with the object that comes immediately to mind as the companion to antigen—antibody. Antigens call forth a variety of immune responses. Antibody formation is only one of them. It is, however, what we conventionally think of as *the* prime immune entity, and the description of antibody may afford the easiest entry into our consideration of the immune system. Later we'll find out where antibodies come from but first let us consider what they are and what they do.

The papaya has never been my favorite fruit, but it did help win a Nobel Prize. By the 1960s most of the attributes of antibody had been illuminated. It was known that antibody was a serum protein—a globulin-type protein—and that there were five kinds of this protein. The five classes of antibody were labeled *immunoglobulin (Ig)* G, M, A, D, and E. With the exception of IgD, the way in which each of these immunoglobulin antibodies functioned was also pretty well understood. However, the structure of the immunoglobulin molecule and the properties that gave it the ability to attack—to combine with—a specific antigen epitope remained obscure.

Papaya contains an enzyme that breaks down protein (a proteolytic enzyme). You buy this enzyme, papain, prepared and packaged as a meat tenderizer to turn chuck steak into prime porterhouse (in my experience it is more likely to turn it into mushy chuck). What papain does is to act as an enzymatic scissor that cuts the long protein molecule into two shorter (peptide) chains. An immunologist, Dr. Rodney Porter, had the bright idea of pressing papain's cleaving abilities into the service of science. He reasoned that what papain could do for the tough steak-protein molecule it could do for the immunoglobulin molecule, by cutting it into two parts. The function of each part could then be determined. His experiments revealed that one fraction, which he named *Fab*, possessed all the antigen binding activity. The other fraction, which because it could be crystallized he called the *Fc* portion, did not bind antigen. The Fc fraction did however, in the case of the IgG and IgM molecules, have a receptor to bind complement.[3] Porter and other workers then went on to use other proteolytic enzymes that snipped bits and pieces off the antibody protein molecule at sites different than that cleaved by papain. Very-high-resolution electron microscopy was also used to visualize the structure of the immunoglobulin molecules(s). From these techniques a picture of the immunoglobulin

3. Complement is one of the "natural immune" substances in the serum. Complement acts along with antibody to make several important immune reactions, such as the killing and lysing of bacteria, "go." More of complement in Chapter 7.

molecule began to emerge, and for his scientific artistry
Rodney Porter was awarded the Nobel in 1972.

The picture showed that all five classes of immunoglobulins have the same basic structure, which I have illustrated in somewhat stylized fashion (see Figure 1). You will
see that the immunoglobulin molecule has a Y shape made
up of two long chains, each consisting of about 440 amino
acids, bound together by sulfur atoms. Also bound by sulfur atoms to each arm of the Y is a short chain of about 220
amino acids. The long and the short of it to immunologists
is that the long chain is called the *heavy chain,* and the
short chain, the *light chain.* The Fab (antigen-combining)
fraction of the immunoglobulin molecule was found to

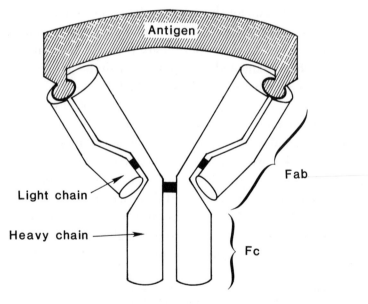

**Figure 1**
THE IMMUNOGLOBULIN MOLECULE: a stylized representation

be the yearning arms of the Y and the Fc portion the "stem."

By snipping off bits and pieces with enzyme "scalpels," together with the modern technology of amino acid sequencing that identified the type and position of each successive amino acid in a protein / peptide chain, it was possible to fill in the fine details of the immunoglobulin picture. The latest portrait of immunoglobulin molecule shows:

1. The antigen (epitope) binding sites on the Fab ($^V$) fraction are confined to an area on the first half of each arm (the variable region). In this variable region the actual sites where the antigen epitope is bound consist of one or more patches of a sequence of six to twenty amino acids along the chain. This neatly conforms to the finding that the antigenic determinant, the epitope, is also made up of a similar number of amino acids. The epitope of several antigens have been analyzed and their molecules reconstructed Tinkertoy-fashion to produce three-dimensional, sculptured models. The antibody to those epitopes has also been obtained, and their "patch" sites that combine with a particular epitope similarly characterized for amino acid composition and sequence and modeled. When the two models—that of the epitope and that of its antibody-combining "patch"—have been put together they have been found to fit together like two matching pieces of a jigsaw puzzle.

2. The amino acid sequence and composition of the Fc segment—the stem of the antibody-immunoglobulin molecule—is constant.

Suppose you had an infection with a *Staphylococcus* bacteria. Your immune system would react by producing an IgG antibody to it (actually, to an epitope of the bacteria antigen). Then suppose a little while later you caught the flu and the immune system produced another IgG antibody, this time to the influenza virus. The variant region of the Fab portion of the two antibodies would have different amino acid composition and sequence because their epitope-combining patches would have to be different. Each would have to have a unique amino acid sequence to give it the configuration that would allow the interlocking with its epitope. However, the Fc portion of both IgG antibodies would have exactly the same amino acid construction.

3. But IgG is not the lone antibody: there are *five* kinds of immunoglobulin and it is the Fc segments that give them the touch of class. IgG, IgM, IgA, IgD, and IgE differ from one another in the composition of their respective Fc's. The number, kinds, and sequence of amino acid making up the immunoglobulin molecule's "stem" lends it a molecular weight and other properties, described later, typical of its class.

4. One final burden of fact about your immunoglobulin molecules. An IgG (as well as each of the other four immunoglobulin classes) of mouse and man are the same—but different. If an IgG from one animal species—say a mouse—were injected into another animal species—say a man—in this case the human would recognize the mouse IgG as foreign (antigenic) and produce an antibody to it: human anti-mouse IgG antibody (and vice versa if human IgG were injected into a mouse).

The immunoglobulins have been around for a long time (more precisely, the genes that code for manufacture of the immunoglobulins have been around for a long time). Recognizable IgM came along with the bony fishes some 300 million years ago. IgG, however, is purely a mammalian invention, a mere 180 million years old—give or take a few years. As each species evolved, their genetic makeup changed. The genes that code for immunoglobulin assembly also altered slightly with the evolution of a species; a substitution of a just a few amino acids, mainly in the Fc segment of the molecule, gave the species its own immunoglobulin signature. For example, the signatures of a mouse's and a rat's IgG are both, patently, IgG molecules. But the slight difference in their amino acid construction would make them foreign—antigenic—in the recipient animal. If IgG from a mouse were injected into a rat, the rat's immune system would detect it as a foreign substance and produce an antibody to it (rat and anti-mouse IgG antibody).

The phenomenon I have just described is more than an esoteric fact of immunochemistry. It has an important bearing on the application and limitations of serotherapy—the treatment of diseases (particularly, infectious diseases) by serum antibodies prepared in laboratory animals. After reading about the treatment of diptheria with antidiptheria serum from immunized horses you might well ask, Why didn't biomedical research pursue that route? Why all the research effort on new drugs and antibiotics to treat infections? It would seem logical to make an antibody in a horse or cow, or any other convenient animal, to whatever germ is going around. Got a strep throat? Why not take a shot of antistrep serum (antibody) produced by a horse-immunizing factory? Another infection? Another shot from a horse of a different antibody.

It's that second horse (antibody) that makes serotherapy impossible as a conventional form of treatment. Remember the diphtheric child given the antitoxic horse serum back in nineteenth-century Berlin? Within minutes after the injection the antibody combined with the toxin and began to neutralize it. However, over the next few days, before the horse serum could be completely cleared from the body, the child's immune system began to recognize it as something alien and started producing an antibody to it (human anti-horse IgG and / or IgM). Now, if our bad-luck child were to have, say, tetanus at a later date and be given antitetnus serum also raised in a horse, the child's antibody would react with the horse serum. Not only would this vitiate the antitoxin action, but the massive, rapid combination of the child's antibody and the horse serum would be harmful, possibly even lethal. Under normal circumstances the body "meters" the immune reactions so that everything proceeds at optimal kinetics. If great amounts of antibody and antigen are brought together by wrongful inoculation or in certain abnormal immunological reactions associated with some diseases, the large amount of immune complexes formed induce serum sickness—immune complex disease—whose symptoms range from fever to a fatal, shock-like (anaphylactic) reaction.

## *The Wizards of Ig—Your Immunoglobulins*

So far a lot has been said about your Ig's without saying anything about what they actually do, other than the general proposition that they combine with antigen. Of course, that is their main function, but they do so in a fashion and place that makes each a class by itself.

### IgM

This is a grand immunoglobulin, and that's not only a figure of speech: IgM is usually the initial immunoglobulin to be produced following the first experience with an antigen. For example, if you had never had malaria before you went to India as a tourist (and forgot to take your antimalaria pills) the first antibody to show up in your blood serum would be an antimalaria (anti-*Plasmodium*) IgM. It is big because it is actually five immunoglobulin molecules bound together in cartwheel fashion (see Figure 2). And, because there are five Y components instead of the single Y of the other immunoglobulin classes, IgM has five times as many antigen binding sites. Thus, theoretically each IgM antibody molecule could inactivate ten bacteria, whereas the IgG antibody molecule would inactivate only two bacteria.

If IgM is all that wonderful then why do we need any other kinds of immunoglobulins? IgM's shortcoming is its short life. All serum proteins are broken down—metabolically decayed—over a period of time and the products recycled as building material of renewal. The body corporate may be entitled to its three score and ten years but for

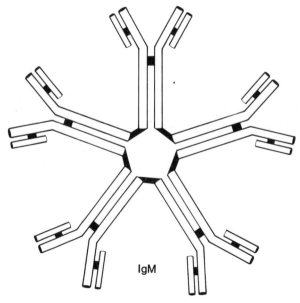

Figure 2

many of its components there is constant death and replacement. A red blood cell lives an average of 120 days; an epithelial cell of the intestinal lining lives 3 days, and the IgM antibody molecule lives only 5 days before being (metabolically) sent to the wreckers. Although the clone of cells that manufacture IgM antibody (the plasma cells— Chapters 6 and 7) expands after antigenic stimulation they don't usually become all that abundant, and this—combined with the short life span of the molecule—does not generally allow IgM antibody levels to be maintained at effectively high levels of concentration in the blood.

### IgG

In the usual course of an immune response—during an infection with a pathogen, for example—IgG is the second type of antibody that appears. If it is the "second time around," such as after reinfection with the same pathogen or after a booster immunization shot, then the IgG antibody would be produced immediately without the IgM preliminaries. Let's go back to your feverish trip to India. You get malaria—not the fatal kind, fortunately. After about four days IgM antibody can be detected in your serum and then some ten days later IgG antibody is present. Suppose you return to India a year later, and again forget to take your pills (you clod!) and get malaria again; in this case IgG antibody, and only IgG antibody, would be detectable in your serum after about three to four days from the time the parasites first appeared in your blood. More of this later in Chapter 7.

IgG (there are four subclasses of IgG but for our purposes they will be considered as being of a single class) may only be a simple Y molecule and bind less antigen (epitope) than IgM but it it is much longer lived—twenty-three to twenty-eight days as compared to the five-day metabolic life span of IgM molecules. Also, the cells that produce IgG antibody are longer-lived than the cells that produce IgM.

IgG is unique, being the only immunoglobulin capable of crossing the placenta from the mother to her unborn child. It is nature's Head Start program. Let us use malaria again as an example of this phenomenon (I happen to be partial to malaria; there are other infectious diseases that would serve equally well). The children living in highly endemic regions experience repeated attacks of malaria. The survivors gradually develop an immunity, and by the time they become young adults there is little in the way of symptomatic infection. A specific IgG antibody acting against the malaria parasite is an essential component of this funcional immunity. Thus, most pregnant women of the Third (malarious) World have this antibody in their blood and it will be transferred to the fetus. When the child is born it will have the antimalaria antibody obtained from the mother in *its* blood, and will be protected from the infection. The protection, however, will only last a month or two since the newborn does not have its own antimalaria immune reaction started up and the passively acquired mother's antibody will be metabolically degraded. Nevertheless, the mother has given her infant an immunological "cover" during the highly vulnerable first months of postnatal life during which the child's immune system is developing to full reactive maturity.

### IgA

IgA is the immunoglobulin of diverse humors—blood, milk, spit, tears, and intestinal juices. The other immunoglobulins, particularly IgG and IgM, are at highest concentration in the blood plasma (they are also present in the liquid that bathes the central nervous system, the cerebro-spinal fluid). IgA is different: it is at low concentration in the blood and at relatively high level in body secretions such as saliva and milk. Like IgM, its molecular life is short—five to six days. Despite this brief life span IgA is important in immunological defense because it gets to sites where the "blood immunoglobulins" IgG and IgM cannot, or do so at low concentrations. It is an antibody of our tracts—gastrointestinal, respiratory, and genitourinary—where it binds to (and inactivates) pathogenic bacteria, their toxins, and viruses.

There was a time not long ago when breast-feeding lost its cachet. It was considered to be less convenient for mother and child than formula, and mother's milk was thought to be no more nutritious than commercial preparations of a cow's-milk base. Not considered was the immune protection afforded by mother's milk, although as long ago as 1892 Paul Ehrlich had shown that newborn mice suckled by mothers that had been vaccinated against bacterial toxins were protected against those toxins. Even so, milk and colostrum (the clear liquid that precedes milk) were not thought to confer a similar immunity.[4] As late as 1958, a pediatrician of high repute was to write in *Advances in Pediatrics* ". . . data refute the concept that human milk is of any appreciable importance of protective antibodies for the child."

4. Veterinarians knew better, but then their patients were cows and horses. The placenta of ruminants does not allow the passage of IgG to the fetus as in humans. Instead, the intestinal wall of ruminants is so constructed as to allow the passage of IgG in the colostrum from the lumen of the gut through the intestinal lining and into small blood vessels and thus into the blood. This passage occurs for only a short period after birth; then the intestine changes so as to be impermeable to further passage of antibody. In humans, of course, this does not occur, the IgG is delivered from mother to her child entirely through the placenta.

We don't believe that today. Although the data derive mainly from epidemiological rather than experimental observations, they are sufficiently persuasive that given the choice mothers should give the breast and not the bottle. Breast-fed infants have significantly lower death and illness rates than formula-fed infants. This is true not only in the Third World, where the benefit of breast-feeding could be attributed to the contaminated water used in making up the formula or the frugal use of an insufficient amount of milk powder; the difference also holds true for industrialized societies.

The reduction in illness afforded by breast-feeding is due to protection against intestinal infections and *that* is mainly due to the antimicrobial IgA antibodies in mother's milk that bathe the intestine. There is also evidence that the breast-fed infant is better protected against respiratory infections. The tentative explanation offered for this is that during suckling some milk (and its IgA) will pass over to the respiratory tract. Still another argument in favor of the nurturing breast is that breast-feeding will protect infants who, by reason of inheritance, are likely to become allergic. The reason for this is not known, but allergy involves IgE antibodies—and I'll move on to that immunoglobulin class next.

### IgE

Hay fever? That's your IgE talking. In normal individuals this immunoglobulin is a very minor constitutent of the blood plasma, about .05 mg per 100 ml of plasma (as compared to IgG, which has an average concentration of approximately 1,000 mg per 100 ml of plasma). Allergic individuals such as hay-fever sneezers and asthmatics have a much higher level of IgE in their blood than normal. Most of the augmented IgE is antibody that reacts with the sub-stances provoking the allergic reaction (I'll elaborate on this shortly).

But it is the parasitic worms that really bring out the IgE. It is not uncommon for a "wormy" person to have a serum IgE level five hundred times greater than normal and even ten to one hundred times greater than an allergic person. The reason or reasons for worms calling forth the production of so much IgE is not clear. There is a theory that the reason may be rooted in the very remote past. We can only assume that the immune system and its mecha-nisms evolved because they were of selective advantage to the species. But the allergic state—an immunological phe-nomenon—makes no adaptive (Darwinan) sense. What benefit can be gained from hay fever, overreacting to a bee sting, or asthma? The "wormists" argue that at some time in mammalian evolutionary development the allergic reac-tion became established for the purpose of giving the par-asites an "asthmatic attack." From man to the platypus all mammalian species have unwelcome worm tenants embed-ded in their intestinal wall. IgE antibody directed against these parasites has been shown experimentally as the agent to give them an eviction notice. We shall see that the union of IgE antibody to its antigen causes the release of hista-mine and other pharmacologically potent substances to be released from certain cells in our body. The metabolic products of the worms act as such antigens, cause hista-mine to be released from the cells in the intestine, and this, in turn, gives the worm an "allergic spasm." The worm "sneezes," releases its hold on the gut, and is swept away in the fecal mass. Thus, when that first mutant IgE-produc-ing cell tentatively produced the first molecules of that immunoglobulin, it may have been selected for perpetuation in man's distant relatives because it was a kind of worm medicine—an anthelmintic. Unfortunately, a good thing became a disaster: IgE-producing cells eventually arose that recognized and responded to all allergy antigens that now bedevil us.[5]

Are all the antigens capable of eliciting IgE antibody and the allergy that goes with it? The answer is a qualified yes. First of all, it is common knowledge that certain things are much more likely to cause allergies than most other things (antigens). For example, pollen, house-dust mites, and (as we have just noted) parasitic worms have great ability to stimulate IgE antibody production. Such antigens are referred to as *allergens*. The molecular acrobatics that makes one antigen an allergen calling forth an IgE antibody and another antigen a non-allergen-eliciting IgG or IgM antibody are not known.

In the second place, the kind of antibody response to a given antigen (other than an allergen) is part of our genetic destiny. Immunoglobulins, like all other proteins, are assembled by the cell's RNA from instructions given by the genetic code, DNA. In the majority of people (the immunological norm), a confrontation with an antigen other than an allergen will bring forth the production of IgM and / or IgG antibody. In some people, however, the genetic code is such that it will direct the assembly of an IgE antibody. These are the people who have an inherited tendency to become allergic. However, while the *tendency* to be allergic is inherited the *specificity* is not. Thus, parents who are, for example, allergic to cat dander will not pass on that

5. A fuller discussion of the relationship between worms and IgE and the rather paradoxical hypothesis that worms may both cause and protect against asthma and other allergic conditions is given in my earlier book *New Guinea Tapeworms and Jewish Grandmothers* in the chapter entitled "The Wheeze and the Worm" (New York: Norton, 1981).

particular sensitivity to their children. Their children will have a greater probability than others of developing an allergy but it will almost always be to something quite different than that which causes their parent's hypersensitivity. The child of the cat-dander-allergic parent may have a tendency to develop sometime during his or her life an immune (IgE) aversion to shrimp, or milk, or house-dust mites, or any of the thousands of potential "environmental" allergens.

IgE is the antibody of allergy because it operates in a different manner than does IgG, IgM, and IgA antibodies. Those antibodies combine directly with the antigen for which they are specific—to the cell wall of a bacterium, or to a toxin or some other soluble antigen in the serum, for example. Not so with IgE. IgE antibody-antigen interactions take place on the membrane surface of basophils and mast cells.[6] The chemical structure of the outer enclosing membrane of these cells is such that there are special sites—receptor sites—at which the Fc portion of the IgE molecule can "dock." Other immunoglobulin classes do not have the configuration that gives them docking privileges at these receptor sites. This is illustrated by Figure 3.

The docking of an IgE antibody molecule at its receptor site on the mast cell or basophil surface membrane does not by itself cause the allergic reaction. For this to happen, two IgE molecules of the same antibody must dock at side-by-side receptor sites. The next required event is that their

6. A basophil is a type of white blood cell (leukocyte) containing blue-staining granules. A mast cell is a fixed (noncirculating) cell present in many different kinds of body tissues. Both of these cells are biogenic bombs loaded with histamine and other chemicals of potential biological activity. Histamine and its related amines cause increased small-blood-vessel permeability, smooth muscle contraction, and other adverse physiologic effects.

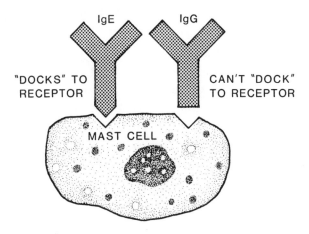

**Figure 3**

allergen must float by and be captured by these molecules in such a way that it forms a bridge across them (Figure 4).

When the bridging occurs, a chemical-energetic signal is sent to the basophil or mast cell to discharge their gran-

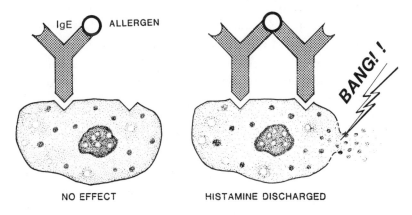

**Figure 4**

ular packets of histamine and other biogenic substances.[7] The effect may be violent but it is really another of nature's immunological strategies for expelling the alien allergen—as it may do for the alien worm. Histamine and the histamine-like substances cause the blood vessels to become leaky—to become more permeable. This partly explains your runny nose, trying to wash away your allergenic demons. These substances also cause smooth muscle contraction—the sneeze, the cough, the wheeze. It is a kind of numbers game: the more IgE antibody and the more allergen, the more histamine is released. And as the hurricane may be of the same meterological lineage as the gentle rains of spring, so too nature's immunological system may overreact. The sneeze of the mild, immediate, hypersensitive response may become the affliction of hay fever and may exaggerate to become the gasping wheeze of asthma.

### IgD

There's not much to be said about IgD: very little is known about its immunological function. It is present in the blood serum at low concentrations, only slightly higher than that of IgE in normal individuals. Like IgE and IgM, IgD has a short metabolic life span of approximately three days. Recently, IgD has been reported as being bound to B lymphocytes. The educated guess / scientific hypothesis is that IgD is involved in specific antigen binding and its

7. There are at least three other substances with a histamine-like action that are released during an allergic episode. These are serotonin, bradykinin, and something called slow-reacting-substance. The antihistamine pill you take acts only against histamine, not against these other biogenic substances. That's why your symptoms may continue after taking the antihistamine.

recognition at the lymphocyte's surface. In some unknown way, this is thought to stimulate the proliferation and maturation of that clone of B cells. (That was all pretty complicated, but don't worry—the crucial role of lymphocytes in the immune response will be more concretely explained in Chapter 7.)

# Chapter 6

# E Pluribus Immunity

ASTROPHYCISISTS possibly excepted, most of us are humbled and fascinated by immensity—the national debt, the stars in the sky, the dimension of eternity. Diversity in the immunological cosmos is of similarly stunning numbers. "Diversity" has already been mentioned as being fundamental to our understanding of the immune system and how it works. So far it's been on the level of "Gee whiz! Look at all the antigens and antibodies!" Scientists have been equally intrigued by this aspect of immunity. As one recent reviewer of the history of immunology, Arthur M. Silverstein, has commented, "the exquisite specificity so characteristic of the immune response has entranced immunologists for 80 years." Theory has succeeded theory as to how the immune system produces an almost infinite number of antibodies in response to an almost infinite number of antigens. The latest, best, and truest theory, *clonal selection*, is the dogma upon which modern immunology rests. I will give an explanation of it and how it evolved so that what follows in the next chapters will be more readily understandable.

Not long after the discovery of antibody, the explanation for diversity and specificity that was advanced said that antibody was not actually formed by the body. This theory held that antibody was merely a fragment of the antigen that had been degraded by a metabolic process. It was believed that this "fragment" could combine with the original whole antigen and this gave it its immunological properties. The theory was untenable because, if a horse was immunized with a diptheria antigen, for example, the same amount of antibody would persist even after the horse had been bled repeatedly. If the antitoxin (antibody) was, in fact, only a break-down product of the antigen used to immunize the horse, then it should have been depleted, diluted, after numerous blood samples had been withdrawn. That the antitoxin level (titre) remained constant indicated that it was being continuously elaborated somewhere, somehow, in the horse's body.

The next explainer was Dr. Ehrlich. Ehrlich proposed that from the surface of the (unknown) antibody-producing cell there sprouted numerous "side chains." Each side chain, the antibody in actuality, was designed to combine with a specific antigen. The theory became a little more fuzzy and mystical with the further proposition that the "side-chain" cell was phagocytic and capable of ingesting the antigen. The cell once it had ingested the antigen responded "with the ancient wisdom of its protoplasm"; it adjusted its metabolism accordingly to produce a shower of the complimentary antigen-specific side chains. At the time, this was a logical hypothesis. It was also consonant with the Darwinian tenets of selection-evolution. Ehrlich's reasoning asserted that the cell had, through evolutionary selection, developed the mechanism to make the side chains (antibodies) against the pathogens and toxins that beset the species and its ancestor. When Ehrlich formulated his side-chain theory this was a reasonable assumption. Only a relatively few antigens had been identified, and they were all of a pathogenic or noxious derivation. However, when a few years

later, it became evident that all sorts of harmless substances could be antigenic the side-chain theory lost its
appeal to reason. The main defect in the theory was that
the cell surface simply couldn't hold all the many million
side chains (specific antibody molecules) complementing all
the many million of possible antigens.

In the 1930s and 1940s the instruction theories were
offered as an answer to the vexing questions posed by antigen and antibody diversity. In those decades, the facts of
life about antibody and genes were just beginning to be
appreciated. It was then known that antibodies were globulin proteins and genes were somehow involved in the
making of those proteins. Where antibodies were made,
the molecular shape that gave the antibodies specificity,
the genetic code, and how the code gave instructions for
protein assembly was knowledge fifteen, or more, years
away. Based on the knowledge of the day, it was proposed
that the (unknown) cell type which produced antibody was
nonspecifically "plastic"—it could be bent to the antigen's
will. The theory agreed with Ehrlich's supposition that this
cell was phagocytic and internalized the antigen. The
departure from Ehrlich was that in the new hypothesis, the
antigen acted as a template to *instruct* the cell to make the
specific, complimentary antibody. How the antigen-tem-
plate actually instructed the cell to make the antibody wasn't
clear. One school held that as yet unidentified enzymes
assembled the globulin proteins and that the antigen somehow modified the enzyme so that it would assemble an
antibody protein to its template mold. Another school of
thought proposed that once the antigen was taken within
the cell it came into contact with the genes in the cell's
nucleus. The antigen, according to this subtheory, instructed

the gene (in some unknown fashion) to make the complimentary antibody protein.

In 1958, Francis Crick promulgated the genetic law that a protein was made by the precoded instruction from the gene's DNA to the RNA. The RNA then assembled the protein. This law, which had the authority of experimental proof, shot down the instructional theory(s) for antibody diversity. The antigen might conceivably *initiate* production, but it did not and could not instruct a "plastic" gene to make an antibody to its specifications. There was no "plastic" gene. The gene was already fixed (unless it mutated). It was already coded, predestined to govern the making of a single antibody type of a single specificity.

Given the foregoing biological facts, there seemed to be only one possible mechanism to account for antibody diversity, clonal selection. This mechanism was so different from any other known process of mammalian life that it was, at first, conceptually difficult to accept. The assumption was correctly made that each antibody-producing cell coded for the making of one antigen-specific antibody: one cell—one antibody. The stunning implication of that premise was that each individual must possess an enormous pool of cells capable, under the appropriate circumstances, of producing antibody(s). Moreover, *each* cell in that individual's pool would produce an antibody of different specificity. This cell would produce an antibody that would combine with a tetanus bacillus only, that cell would produce an antibody that would combine with a pollen antigen only—*ad infinitum*, each cell to its own antigenic Mr. Right. This pool of diverse, antibody-producing cells was shown to be, for each of us, our immunogenetic inheritance. *We are born* with all the cells that will elicit an antibody to every antigen there is, or ever will be. Mutations are thought to expand the pool's potential even further and the present estimate is that mouse and man (and presumably all other mammals) have within them the means to produce anywhere from 10 billion to 100 billion different kinds of antibodies. Stupendous!

This brings us to part II of the clonal selection theory. Obviously, there aren't 10 to 100 billion cells vigorously producing 10 to 100 billion antibodies. Our blood would soon become oversaturated with immunoglobulins. Nature isn't that inefficient. (However, in 1955 the Danish immunologist Niels Jerne published a paper in which he proposed that small amounts of antibodies of all possible specificities actually existed in the blood. There has been no convincing experimental evidence to confirm that theory.) To microbiologists and tissue-culture experts the way antibodies were produced "as needed" was quite simple. It was accomplished by an expansion of a clone. If, by some fancy manipulation, you isolated a *single* bacterium or any other kind of passionless cell that divides asexually[1] and put that cell into a suitable growth medium, the cell would divide repeatedly to develop into a population of cells. And, because they derived asexually from a single cell, each cell of that population would be identical to the parent cell and to each other. By definition, they would be a clone. In 1957, the Australian biologist-microbiologist-physician Sir Macfarlane Burnet brought all these observations together to present a closely reasoned argument for the clonal selection theory of antibody diversity. This theory, which Burnet is given credit for formulating, has since been elaborated

1. There are no male or female genetic contributors to cells that reproduce asexually. In these cells, such as an ameoba or epithelial cell of our intestinal lining, the nucleus genetic material (chromosomes) simply splits into two identical portions—divides—and then the cell cytoplasm divides to form two *identical* daughter cells.

upon and continues to be "fleshed out" by new experimental findings.

There are still a good many gaps in the clonal selection theory, especially as they relate to the dynamics responsible for the sequence of events that causes the clone to expand and the antibody to be produced. However, it has passed from theory to acceptance as the proven mechanism responsible for antibody diversity. We shall get a better idea how it all works in Chapter 7, but synoptically the theory propounds:

1. We are all born with a pool of cells (now known to be *B lymphocytes*—Chapter 7); each cell in the pool has the potential to produce an antibody of singular specificity.

2. When an antigen is introduced into the body it eventually unites with that single cell (lymphocyte) in the pool for which it is specific. It is an exclusive union.

3. The union of antigen with its lymphocyte "ignites" a reaction in the lymphocyte, which causes it to divide repeatedly. Consequently, a large population, a clone, of that cell line is formed.

4. The cells (lymphocytes) in that clone mature and begin producing the antibody specific for the antigen.

Thus we are born with a wonderful endowment of immune capacity. No one is quite certain how we came by it but it seems to have been in place a long, long time—at least since the ancient mammals. In the next chapter we shall go on to learn something more about how it operates.

# Chapter 7

# The Immune System Turns On, Continued: T Cells and B Cells

THIRTY years ago immunology was a relatively simple, eminently understandable discipline. Phagocytes devoured foreign particulate matter such as bacteria, while specific antibody (produced by some unknown cell line) combined with and inactivated bacteria and all other particulate and nonparticulate foreign matter (the antigens). It was also known that there was a kind of immune memory in that a second shot of vaccine or a second exposure to a pathogenic microbe resulted in accelerated production, and a greater amount of antibody, than after the primary antigenic experience.

Thirty years later, phagocytes still devour bacteria and antibodies still bind to the antigens which evoked them. What is different is our understanding of these phenomena. Immunological research carried out during the intervening years has revealed these immune responses to be endgame plays of a complex series of cellular interactions.

The New Immunology began in the mid-1950s with studies on two bits of internal anatomy whose function was then unknown and considered by some scientists as useless relics of evolution—the bursa of Fabricius (a lymph node–

like structure attached to the cloaca[1] of birds), and the thymus gland.[2] Early twentieth-century (pre-1950s) experimentalists had approached the problem of determining what
these anatomical structures did in a subtractive manner.
Cut it out, sew the experimental animal back up, and wait
to see what happens. Nothing happened.

The report that was to change our concept of immunity
so radically did not appear in a journal frequented by the
scientific illuminati, such as the *Journal of Experimental
Medicine*, but as a two-page research note in a "bird mag-
azine," *Poultry Science*. A young graduate student at the
University of Ohio, Bruce Glick, chose the riddle of the
bursa of Fabricius as his dissertation topic. Up to that time,
the extirpation experimenters had used adult or juvenile
animals since they were more convenient to operate on than
young animals. Glick did something different: during the
course of his doctoral research he removed the bursa from
very young birds. This had no discernible effect and the
birds were put in a cage and pretty well forgotten. A year
later, in 1956, the now Dr. Glick was at the Ohio Agricultural Experimental Station and had need of antibody against
a bacteria of birds, *Salmonella typhimurium*. To get the
antibody he and his colleagues, Timothy Chang and George
Jaap, did much the same thing as Pasteur had done by chance
almost a hundred years before. They inoculated the birds

1. Birds have no separate urogenital and intestinal tracts emptying to
the outside. The urogenital duct leads within the body, into the lower
gut. A chicken defecates, lays an egg, and urinates through a common
tube—the cloaca. Efficient but not neat and so the name—*cloaca*, Latin
for "sewer."

2. Because it gradually atrophies after puberty the thymus gland, a
"sweetbread" lying in the anterior of the chest, was for many years thought
to have no function—a vestigial relic inherited from the dinosaurs like
that other bit of useless tissue, the appendix.

with an oldish culture of the bacteria. Quite by accident, among the birds inoculated there happened to be some that Glick had bursectomized the year before, which had now grown to adults. These birds—like *les poulets de* M. Pasteur—should have become immunized, antibodied, and remained healthy. Not so Dr. Glick's *poulets*. Some died. Most produced little or no antibody. To Glick et al.'s astonishment, when they went back to the records all the dead and antibody-less birds were those that had been bursectomized as chicks. The experiment was repeated and the same results obtained. When adult birds were bursectomized and injected with the *Salmonella* antigen they remained healthy and produced antibody in normal fashion. In this way it came to be realized that the bursa of Fabricius was profoundly involved in the *maturation* of the immune system—particularly in its ability to produce antibody.

About the same time that Bruce Glick was taking the bursa out of baby birds, a physician-immunologist at the University of Minnesota, Dr. Robert Good, was trying to find out what the thymus was doing. He too was an experimental extirpationist. If the organ confuses you, pluck it out. Like the workers who had pursued the bursa of Fabricius' function he found that there was little effect after the thymus was removed from adult animals. Glick's paper in *Poultry Science* came to Good's attention and he decided to try a similar approach—surgical removal of the thymus from newborn mice. Again, this proved the way that was to give the first insight into thymic function—and with that insight came an entirely new view of immunity. Thymectomy of the newborn resulted in a very defective immune system, very similar to that observed for the bursectomized chicks. The mice produced little or no antibody after inoculation with most antigens and they were also tardy in rejecting skin transplants from other animals.

Mice don't have a bursa of Fabricius. Only birds have a bursa. Was the thymus an organ that had taken over the immunological duties of the bursa during the course of evolution from bird to mammal? Probably not. For one thing, birds have a bursa *and* a thymus. The chicken, therefore, had great potential as an experimental animal because either one or both organs could be removed. By 1962, Noel Warner and Alexander Szenberg in Australia, and Max Cooper in Good's laboratory in Minnesota, exploiting this selective surgical technique, were able to report that indeed the bursa and the thymus were responsible for different immunological functions.

The revolutionary idea to flow from this work was that there was more to the immune system than had met the eye for the past fifty years. Up to that time, Ehrlich's theory on the origin of antibody held sway. His theory maintained that there was a specialized type of cell that manufactured antibody (in 1960 the "mother-of-antibody" cell had not yet been identified). The theory went on to hypothesize that antigen acted as a die which *instructed* the cell to make a template antibody to it (as we have already noted, the die and template-instructional theory has now been discarded). From the studies on the thymus and bursa the New Immunologists now proposed that antibody production was not as straightforward as Ehrlich had envisaged it to be. The evidence now pointed to at least two different types of "specialist" cells necessary to produce antibody. One type that recognized the "foreignness" of an antigen and captured it. This recognition cell, it seemed, then passed the information on to the second specialist, which actually produced the antigen-specific antibody of one immunoglobulin class. The thymus was involved with the cells that "recognized" the antigen, while the bursa seemed to be the organ that was involved with the antibody-producing cells.

At that early stage of the investigations the exact identity of those cells wasn't known, but there was a good guess as to what they might be—lymphocytes, the white blood cells with a round nucleus. Both the thymus and the bursa are what histologists call *lymphoid tissue* because they are packed with lymphocytes (the tonsils and lymph nodes are other examples of lymphoid tissue). In 1960, the doings and uses of lymphocytes were as mysterious as they had been since they were first described. For over a hundred years the lymphocyte circulated in blood and lymph in a kind of intellectual limbo. No one had any idea as to its function. I unearthed the histology textbook I had used as a student in the late 1940s and of lymphocytes it says ". . . among their probable functions some connection with fat metabolism and immunity. . . ." As late as 1956 another authoritative text described the lymphocyte as a "somewhat inconspicuous cell with no particularly striking functional or morphological characteristics of its own."

Suspicions of the lymphocyte's role in the immune response were not enough. What were now needed were new methodologies to isolate the lymphocytes from blood and lymphoid tissue, then to maintain them in a viable condition in a culture medium, then to turn them on with antigens and other stimulating agents (mitogens)[3]—and then to

3. Antigens, as will be described, stimulate their specific lymphocytes to mature and proliferate. There are substances, mostly from plants, that turn on all lymphocytes. The health of lymphocytes—and thus the health of the immune system—can be examined by the response of lymphocytes to these substances (mitogens).

be able to measure and characterize any response with an exquisite degree of sensitivity. That's a lot of new technology, but by the mid-1960s all the required methods were in place.

Immunologists could now obtain lymphocytes from an immunized animal and add them to a culture medium containing the antigen used for the immunization. Under these experimental conditions dramatic changes occurred to the antigen-stimulated lymphocytes. They began to grow in size, acquire more cytoplasm and, most significantly, began rapidly to divide resulting in a prodigious increase in their number. Some went on to develop into *plasma cells*.

Plasma cells? In the Chapter 5 the promise was made to tell you where antibodies come from. They come from plasma cells. Plasma cells are larger than lymphocytes (from which they arise), and have a single round nucleus and an abundant cytoplasm. The genetic code of DNA in the plasma cell's nucleus instructs the RNA in the cytoplasm how to assemble an immunoglobulin molecule of a particular class and antibody specificity. That antibody is secreted, at the rate of thousands of Ig molecules a minute, into the blood plasma.

However, of all the "turned-on" lymphocytes in the culture, only a portion transformed into antibody-manufacturing plasma cells. The remaining lymphocytes transformed and they divided repeatedly—but they didn't make immunoglobulin. It was reasoned, therefore, that although all lymphocytes look alike under the microscope, they actually were of two distinct types: one which could, when appropriately stimulated with antigen, become an antibody-secreting cell; and a second type which could also transform and probably do something, but what?

The two kinds of lymphocytes were so outwardly identical that they couldn't be distinguished one from the other by conventional staining and microscopical examination. If further progress was to be made, methods had to be devised to identify each class of lymphocyte and separate it as a simon-pure isolate. This wasn't a theoretical impossibility because if functional differences exist there must be accompanying specifically-different characteristics—biochemical, antigenic, substructural, etc. It didn't take long before these characteristic markers were identified. The lymphocytes that were destined to become immunoglobulin (antibody)-secreting plasma cells were found to have a coating of immunoglobulin bound to their surface. These precursors of the plasma cells made just enough immunoglobulin to envelop themselves and to announce to the rest of the immune system that, given the opportunity, this was that they would manufacture when and if they transformed. Sensitive serological techniques were already available to detect immunoglobulins adherent to cells and other particles, so identifying the pre-plasma lymphocytes by reason of their coat was not difficult.

Finding the marker(s) for the "other" lymphocytes also proved to be a "piece of cake," although methodologically it was a rather odd piece of cake. The observation was made that when lymphocytes from humans or rodents were mixed with the red blood cells of sheep the "other" lymphocytes and only the "other" lymphocytes (they knew that they were the "other" because they didn't have immunoglobulin on their surface) would adhere to the red cells to form a pet-allike pattern—a rosette. Then it was found that if a mixture of lymphocytes was passed through nylon "wool," the "other" lymphocytes would flow through whereas the immunoglobulin-coated, pre–plasma cell lymphocytes would stick to the nylon. I have no idea what prompted anyone to mix lymphocytes with sheep red blood cells or filter them through a tangle of nylon threads. Researchers do some strange things and call it science—and sometimes it is. More recently some very sensitive methods have been devised (monoclonal antibody techniques—to be elaborated on in the final chapter) to characterize the different types and, as it turned out, subtypes of lymphocytes.

When the "marker" techniques became available it was then possible to return to the problems raised by the "extirpation" experiments. What was going on in the thymus and the bursa of Fabricius? Were the two types of lymphocytes somehow related, in some specific way, to these two organs?

These questions could be resolved only by tracing where lymphocytes come from, where they go in the body, and what type they are (or become) when they get there. Studies performed on a series of human embryos revealed that lymphocytes are formed very early in fetal life, arising in the liver by the sixth week of gestation. By the eighth week of fetal life the lymphocytes have departed from the liver to seed the bone marrow. The liver now closes down as a lymphocyte production unit.

In the 1960s, methods were devised to "bell the lymphocyte" in its bone marrow nest with radioactive tracers. This made it possible to follow the lymphocyte in its travels after disseminating from the bone marrow. It was not unlike marking the migration of a whale with an implanted radio transmitter. In this manner it was shown that, although all lymphocytes are created seemingly equal in the bone marrow, they must go to a "vocational school" if they are to become T or B cells.

T and B cells? Beginning early in gestational life (about the tenth week for the human fetus) some lymphocytes migrate from the bone marrow to the thymus. There, under the influence of certain hormones secreted by the thymus, they become the "other" lymphocytes—those without immunoglobulin on their surface—and do not go on to become antibody-secreting plasma cells. Now we can call them by their right name, *T lymphocytes,* or, in immuno-logical parlance, *T cells.*

In birds, conversion to the "antibody" lymphocytes was found to take place in the bursa of Fabricius. The short-hand of science gave the title of *B lymphocytes* or *B cells* to the pre–plasma cell, immunoglobulin-coated lymphocytes. Humans and other mammals do not have a bursa and their B cell "finishing school" organ is not known with any degree of certainty (except that such an organ or collection of tissue must exist). There is some evidence that the mammalian bursal analog is a collection of lymphoid tissue in the intes-tine known as *Peyer's patches.* Other workers are of the opinion that it is the bone marrow itself that creates the B lymphocytes. The bone marrow theory advocates point out that B lymphocytes can already be found in the bone mar-row, blood, and certain other tissues of the twelve-week-old human embryo.

Ten years after Dr. Glick took the bursa out of the chicken and Dr. Good took the thymus from the mouse, the experimental stage was set for an explosive expansion of knowledge that continues to accumulate with each pass-ing day.

It was the T cell that almost immediately following its discovery became the immunologists' darling. It was the new girl in town with moves and features the likes of which had never been seen before. The T lymphocyte resembles the B cell in that it responds in an antigen-specific manner. For each antigen (epitope) there is a T lymphocyte Mr.

Right bearing a mirror-image receptor on its cell membrane surface. And, like the B cell response, the union of antigen to its T cell receptor causes the lymphocyte to proliferate and become functional—to expand the clone. Also like the B cell, the antigen-activated T lymphocyte manufactures and then secretes protein molecules. The big difference is that the secretions of the T cell are not immunoglobulins but a group of proteins called *lymphokines*. Lymphokines may be evoked by a specific interaction of antigen and its T lymphocyte, but unlike immunoglobulin antibodies they do not combine with the antigen (epitope) that stimulated their manufacture. Instead, lymphokines have a repertoire of immunoregulatory functions. For example, if life's abrasions had dealt you an infected big toe, the T lymphocytes (really the expanded clone) responding to the offending bacteria's antigen would begin to secrete a lymphokine. This lymphokine would act as a chemical signal to the phagocytes that they should rally at the infected site. Once the phagocytes had responded to that call, the T lymphocyte would emit another lymphokine[4] which would act to keep the macrophages corralled—to keep them at the focus of infection where they are needed.

Let us now suppose that instead of an infected big toe you are dealt a virus infection—a cold or flu virus, for example. Again, a T cell lymphokine comes to the rescue, only now it is a lymphokine called *gamma interferon*.

Interferon was the explanation of a virologist's problem. Bacteriologists can grow most of their wee beasties in broths and on nutrient agars. Virologists, on the other hand, have a more difficult technical row to hoe. Viruses must, abso-

---

4. The actual number of different kinds of lymphokines hasn't been determined to any degree of certainty. Nor is it known whether or not any one lymphokine has multiple functions.

lutely must, reside within a host cell (they are obligate intracellular parasites) if they are to survive, replicate, and grow. Thus, to maintain a "test-tube" stock of a virus it is first necessary to have a cell line of a tissue that will grow indefinately in a nutrient medium (remember Dr. Alexis Carrel's "immortalized" chicken-heart-cell line that made news in the 1930s).The next step is to get your virus to grow in that cell line. It's a finicky, painstaking business to match your virus with the suitable cell line. And while there is a considerable "library" of viruses that is maintained this way, there are viruses for which the match has never been made. Those viruses must be passaged in experimental animals, if a susceptible animal is available.

Virologists had, for many years, been perplexed that it was difficult or impossible to superimpose a second virus in an already virus-infected tissue culture. They also knew that after a time the virus had to be passaged to a fresh tissue culture, because they stopped invading new cells. As an example of this problem let us imagine that Dr. X wanted to study, in a tissue-culture model, what might happen to a human that was first infected with virus $Y$ and shortly thereafter was also exposed to virus $Z$. He already knows that both $Y$ and $Z$ viruses will grow prolifically in a certain cell line, such as one originating from a monkey kidney. He infects his tissue culture with virus $Y$, which "takes" (that is, he can see clear areas, "plaques," where the virus has destroyed its host cells), and a few days later he would add virus $Z$ to the tissue culture. Under these experimental conditions virus $Z$ failed to invade the tissue-culture cells and become established. There was no secondary infection.

In 1957, two virologists, A. Isaacs and J. Lindemann, finally discovered the cause for the problem that had perplexed and vexed their colleagues. Isaacs and Lindemann started with the supposition that something was being secreted into the nutrient medium by the virus-infected cells of the tissue culture and that something was a factor that either killed the virus or prevented them from invading new host cells. To prove this, they collected the nutrient liquid from a virus-infected tissue culture. This was passed through a filter so fine in pore size that it excluded the passage of any virus that happened to be in the liquid. Next, the filtered, virus-free nutrient was used as an overlay for a passage of the tissue-culture line that had not yet been infected with a virus. The cells of the tissue culture continued to grow normally, so it was concluded that there wasn't anything present that was adversely inhibiting the tissue culture's metabolism or ability to replicate.

The final experimental step was to provide the information that solved the Mystery of the Inhibited Virus. They added the supernatant (overlying liquid) to a "clean" tissue culture and found that when they did this it was impossible to establish viral growth in those cells. The virus failed to "take." It wasn't antibody in the supernatant that was killing the virus. The infected cells were secreting an unusual substance, which didn't actually kill the virus but changed the surrounding cells in such a way as to render them impervious to viral invasion. Isaacs and Lindemann dubbed this factor *interferon*. It was subsequently shown that there are three major classes of interferon, each secreted by a different kind of virus-infected cell: alpha interferon from white blood cells with a lobed nucleus (polymorphonuclear leucocytes); beta interferon from fibroblast cells (supportive, connective, reparative cells); and gamma interferon[5]

5. Gamma interferon can also be obtained from lymphocyte cultures that are not virally infected but stimulated with a variety of strange substances called mitogens. One such mitogen is phytohemagglutinin, which is derived from the red kidney bean, *Phaseolus vulgaris*.

from T lymphocytes. Like all interferons, gamma interferon acts against a multitude of viruses. It also acts against tumor cells, inhibiting their proliferation, and also stimulates certain cells of the immune system to even greater activity.

As you are undoubtedly aware, interferon has been highly publicized as a new kind of biologic wunderkind for the treatment of cancers and viral infections. Unfortunately, in clinical trials it has yet to live up to its good press. Interferon may, indeed, become a powerful therapeutic agent once the problem of preparing sufficient amounts of pure, stable gamma interferon from lymphocyte cultures to undertake meaningful clinical trials has been solved. Recently, the interferon-coding gene has been isolated and inserted into yeast cells and the bacterium *Escherichia coli.* These genetically engineered microorganisms are now beginning to churn out gamma interferon, and clinical trials using this recombinant product are in the planning and early prosecution stages. Curiously, as I write this the white-noise background of my newspeak radio station announces that a commercial interferon nose-drop product is about to be released upon the public to halt the common cold at its first sniffle.

Further research revealed that the "newness" of the T lymphocyte didn't stop at the lymphokines. In the late 1960s it was discovered there wasn't *a* T lymphocyte but, rather, several distinct classes of T lymphocytes, each class having its own unique immunoregulatory function. These T cells were, in fact, the cell types that commanded the cell-soldiers in the trenches—the B lymphocytes and the macrophages—to attack or not to attack, and to inform them that the war had been won and they could now retire to reserve status.

That B lymphocytes didn't do it all alone was first sus-
pected when pure cultures of B lymphocytes taken from an
immunized animal failed to transform into antibody-producing cells as expected after the immunizing antigen was
added to the test-tube culture. However, under these same
experimental conditions, the B cells transformed when T
lymphocytes were also added. Obviously, the B cells needed
a little help from their T cell friends—friends who came to
be called *helper T cells.*

Then another type of T cell was identified, and with its
discovery, the immune system's constitution was discerned
to be, like that of our republic, one of checks and balances.
When certain T cells, particularly those obtained from an
animal during the late curative period of an infection, were
added to B cell cultures, the B cells not only didn't "turn
on" but actually "switched off" their activity if they were
already "turned on" by antigen or mitogen stimulation.
It was these T lymphocytes that said "Stop! Enough already!" and they were, therefore, designated as *suppressor
T cells.*[6]

Actually, it is not quite that straightforward. In order
for both helper and suppressor to start up their antigen-
specific immunoregulatory activities, phagocytes must also
be present. Not only must they be present, they must come
from the same individual that the T cells come from, or
from an identical twin, or—in the case of experimental animals such as mice—from a highly inbred strain (which is

6. If allowed to do so, the clones of B cells and helper T cells—once
transformed by their response to a specific antigen—would keep on pro-
liferating and producing antibodies or lymphokines. This uninhibited,
inappropriate, continuous overmultiplication of a cell type meets the
definition of a cancer. In fact, cancers of the immune system, such as
lymphomas and leukemias, do occur. Hence the necessity of the suppressor T cell in regulating the immune processes.

tantamount to every animal being each other's identical twin). This is by way of saying that all the interreacting cells must be of the same tissue type. Now let us walk through a modified scenario of the immune reaction, again using our infected big toe as the *mise en scène*.

In the beginning there are the phagocytes—early warriors—that wander into the infected site and smite and take into themselves the bacteria. The bacteria are semidigested into several discrete antigenic components by the macrophage's enzymes. These antigenic fragments (epitopes) are transported to the outer surface of the phagocyte's enveloping cell membrane where they are proferred to the helper T lymphocytes that have also infiltrated to the inflamed big toe. One of the helper T cells will be specific for the proferred epitope: it will have a mirror-image receptor site on its membrane that allows for specific binding. The phagocyte[7] and the T cell have yet to be caught *in flagrante delicto* by the immunologist, but somehow they do tryst in order that the epitope can be transferred. However, before the transfer of epitope (a fragment of bacterial antigen, in our case) can take place, the two cells must ask each other "Are you me?" The password for mutual recognition is encoded on their respective outer membranes as specific structural determinants that have been assembled under the direction of a complex of genes. Collectively, these determinants are known as the *major histocompatability complex (MHC)*. The MHC is a determinant of cell type much like the ABO determinants on the red blood cell

7. *Phagocyte* is used here as a convenient descriptive. Not all phagocytes process and present antigen to the T cell. Polymorphonuclear leukocytes, for example, are not "presenting" phagocytes, whereas monocytes and macrophages are.

membrane, but it is a much more complex system than blood type factors in that there are at least twenty-two to twenty-five (and possible several hundred) MHC types. Since we each bear two determinants—one inherited from each parent—and there are some twenty-two different determinants, our HL-A system is, individualistically, highly diverse.[8]

Assuming that the MHC password has been given to the phagocyte's satisfaction it will pass the epitope to the surface of the helper T cell. The underlying mechanisms are not fully understood, but these two events—major histocompatability complex type recognition and antigen transfer—energize the helper T lymphocyte and transform it into a protein-secreting cell. This protein is the "helper factor" and is specific in that it only helps B lymphocytes who have already helped themselves by selectively binding the antigen / epitope to their surface membrane (the specific immunoglobulin on the B cell membrane). Sandwich-fashion, the helper factor binds to the antigen epitope—in this case a snippet of the bacteria in our sore toe—which is bound to the B cell surface. The final layer to the sandwich (the helper T cell factor) causes the B cell to divide repeatedly and transform into a clone of plasma cells secreting a specific antibody.[9] There are a few antigens, mostly polysaccharides of bacterial cell walls, that do not have to go through the phagocyte–T cell–B cell transfer. These anti-

8. MHC matching is of crucial importance in organ transplants. If the immune system recognizes the MHC determinants on the donor's tissues as being different from theirs, they will treat that tissue as an antigen—a foreign body—and attempt to destroy it by antibody and other means just as surely as if it were an invading parasite.

9. "E pluribus immunity" again. It is not certain whether or not there are four B cell lines for each antigen / epitope: one that will produce an

gens act directly on the B cell without any intermediaries.

So now there is antibody to kill the bacteria and begin the curative process, and what a complicated business it has been to get that antibody produced! But as complex as that was, there is more. Nature has provided a feedback that accelerates the curative process still further. During the first few days of the infection the macrophages have been capturing the bacteria in a random, rather sluggish, fashion. The macrophage has been instrumental in processing the antigen to make the humoral (antibody) reaction go forward, but as a devouring instrument of destruction it hasn't been all that efficient. Several factors now urge the macrophages and monocytes to a higher level of activity. To a large extent, contemporary research has confirmed Élie Metchnikoff's view of the macrophage as the true hero of the Immune Wars. It is now realized that many immune responses are directed to amplifying macrophage activity. A T cell lymphokine-,macrophage-activating factor is one such energizer. Antibody also helps. An antigen that has antibody bound to it is much more delectable to the macrophage than an "uncoated" antigen. (This "buttering" of the antigen by antibody is known as *opsonization.*)

So antibody and angry macrophages (with maybe a little discreet assistance from an antibiotic) have cured the big toe. We can once again kick the football for a sixty-yard field goal, get up on point and dance Swan Lake, walk the dog—whatever our ambulatory pursuits may be. Now it is time for the immune reaction to shut down. The signals

---

IgM antibody, one an IgG antibody, another for IgA antibody, and a fourth for IgE antibody. It is known that in some instances a plasma cell will start out making IgM antibody to an antigen and then switch to producing IgG antibody to that antigen.

that switch on the suppressor arm of the immune system have not been clearly defined. At our present state of understanding we can observe end effects of the circuitry—as if they were lights turned on or motors running—but the source of the power input and the wiring diagram itself are rather vaguely comprehended. From mouse experiments, it appears that when antigen (and, probably, antibody) concentrations increase, suppressor T lymphocytes become activated. Also, the news from the mouse is that for several large antigen molecules, which are composed of several epitope determinants, some of those epitopes will induce helper T cell induction and proliferation, while other epitopes of the molecular chain will set the suppressor T lymphocytes loose. We have already seen that it is the macrophage that digestively separates the antigen's molecular chain into its epitope components and presents those epitopes to the T cells. Perhaps it is an "all-wise" macrophage that staggers presentation of epitopes for successive recognition first by helper cells and then by suppressor cells.

Whatever the mechanism, at some point during our big toe's tribulations the suppressor T cell will arrive on the scene and like its helper counterpart will begin to proliferate and mature into a secreting entity. There appears to be multiple suppressor factors: some turn off helper T cell function, some shut down antibody production. Still other factors, elaborated by the suppressor T lymphocyte, act broadly and nonspecifically, irrespective of the antigen / epitope which prompted the "turn on" in the first place.

We lack a clear understanding as to how the suppressor T lymphocytes are themselves suppressed–turned off. Obviously, it would be just as bad, if not worse, to have a continuously dampened immune system as it would be to have a continuously hyperactive one. Recent research has hinted at the presence of a special gene in the lymphocyte's nucleus that codes for the production of a shutdown factor.[10] Presumably, the gene in the T cell nucleus which is orchestrating all this activity somehow "knows" when it is the proper time for it to become activated. The vast majority of T cells (of both types) are relatively short-lived, surviving only three to four days, and thus after shutdown the immune reaction will gradually come to a halt (remember, even the "long-lived" IgG antibody molecule will metabolically decay in about thirty days).

However, if lymphocyte life is so ephemeral, what can explain a central dogma of immunology, "Things go better the second time around"? If, after a suitable interval, one encounters the same antigen again, the immune response is both more vigorous and accelerated than the debut response. This is the reason for the booster shots of immunization—to prime the immunological pump. It is also the reason why the symptoms are milder and of shorter duration during subsequent infections with many, but not all, pathogens.

The reason for this vigorous secondary immune response is that not all the lymphocytes die within a few days of being transformed by antigenic stimulation. A very few antigen-transformed lymphocytes become, in some unknown way, very long-lived cells known as *memory B* and *memory T* cells. These Peter Pan lymphocytes continue to circulate in the blood or "hibernate" in a lymphoid organ such as the

10. There is also evidence that yet another subset of T cells may be involved in the final closedown of the immune reaction. These have been labeled *contra suppressor T cells.* An immunologist friend who brought this to my attention assures me that there are no Central American political implications in the name.

spleen until they are again restimulated with the specific antigen. When this occurs the memory cells proliferate very rapidly to become populous clones of functioning helper T cells and / or antibody-secreting B cells (plasma cells). In some respects our immunological memory has a greater capacity for recall than does our brain.

## *Doctor Frankenstein Meets the Killer T Cell*

The account so far would have it that the lymphocytes who play the endgame of attacking specific antigen targets are all B cells whose weapons are the humors of immunity—immunoglobulin antibody. Now I must introduce (believe me, reluctantly) still another class of lymphocyte activists: T lymphocytes, who play the endgame and do so without the means of antibody—the cytotoxic killer T cells.

It may be that Dr. Frankenstein's assembled creature and the Six Million Dollar Man continue to seize our imagination because they represent humanity's deep-seated wish to replace their aging and damaged limbs and organs with "factory fresh" parts. Surgeons have, to a large extent, developed the techniques and skills to make many of the transplantation hookups but the dream of replacing flesh with flesh, limb with limb, organ with organ remains largely unfulfilled. That failure is more immunological than technical in cause.

Skin transplantation has long been an objective of research. The ultimate beneficiaries would mainly be burn victims who often require extensive skin replacement. Moreover, a skin transplant is, technically, relatively easy to do and thus lends itself to experimental study. For example, a patch of skin from a black mouse can be patched onto a white mouse in order to follow the fate of the transplant.

However, none of the experimental attempts have been successful except when the donor and the recipient were of the same highly inbred strain of mouse. Otherwise, the grafted skin began to die after about a week, and within two weeks was completely dead. If the recipient mouse was given a second skin graft several weeks later the rejection process was even more rapid, usually within three to four days.

When, in these early studies, a bit of tissue was taken from the junction of the recipient's skin and the dying graft an infiltration of lymphocytes could be seen. But since at that time the function(s) of the lymphocyte was unknown, the meaning of their presence at the dying graft site was also unknown. As is so often the case in solving a problem through "orderly" research, the demystification of rejection did not proceed in logical order. The process of discovery reads more like the plot of a mystery novel. First there is the killing, after which the killer and his *modus operandi* are described. However, in the current edition of our mystery the detective-immunologists are still not satisfied as to the nature of the actual weapon and whether or not the killer has any accomplices.

The story opens in 1960 with the report by Dr. A. Govaerts in the *Journal of Immunology.* Govaerts had harvested the lymphocytes from the lymphatic fluid and lymphatic glands of a dog which had rejected an experimentally transplanted kidney. He washed the lymphocytes to free them from lymphatic fluid, resuspended them in culture medium and then added kidney cells from the donor dog to the culture. To his surprise, Govaerts observed that in the presence of these lymphocytes the kidney cells were not only killed rapidly but they were also lysed (dissolved)—as if they had been put in a bath of strong acid or digestive juices. This was very peculiar because there was no reason—no known immunological motive—for the death of the kidney cells. Antibody in the presence of complement could kill and lyse the targeted kidney cell. But there was no antibody in Govaerts's experimental system. Macrophages could kill targeted cells but would not lyse them until they had been ingested. This was a new phenomenon involving a hitherto unknown type of lymphocyte—a cytotoxic killer lymphocyte.

We have already noted that the 1960s was a decade of rapidly advancing research on the lymphocyte. It was a time when the lymphocyte classes and their functions were beginning to be elucidated. Each type of lymphocyte was shown to carry a characteristic surface marker—in effect, a unique antigenic character by which they could be identified. When the "marker" tests were applied to the cytotoxic lymphocyte it was found that it was a member of the T cell family but differed in several subtle respects from its helper and suppressor cell relatives.

So here was a very different T cell; all the other T cells were entrepreneurs acting as the middlemen of the immune responses. The cytotoxic T cell was very different not only because it was an endgame player but also because it exerted its effect in a manner that differed from all other lymphocytes. All the other lymphocytes seem to act at a distance from their target cells by means of their chemical signals. The B cells secrete antibodies, whereas helper and suppressor T cells secrete helper and suppressor factors. From what is known of the cytotoxic T cell it appears that it must get close to its target, actually make contact with it, in order to kill. Its instrument of lethality is unknown but it seems to be a chemical one that destroys the target cell's enveloping membrane. In that deadly encounter the cytotoxic T cells survive and go on to kill again. The means by which it can destroy the target cell membrane while its own membrane remains unaffected is not known.

The main targets of cytotoxic T cells are viruses and "foreign" major histocompatability complex antigens (as would exist on the surface of cells in a mismatched organ transplant). Thus, the major immunological activities of these militants are (1) to defend against invading viruses, and (2) to kill cells bearing a major histocompatability antigen different from its own (graft rejection is the most notable example of this activity). The action is a specific one, directed against specific antigen targets. It also appears that the cytotoxic T cells are called forth by accomplice cells, macrophages, and inducer T cells—a complicated process that is best left to students of immunology.

I noted earlier that when a second graft from the same donor is put in place, that graft is rejected much more quickly than the first. The presence of antibody and a second round of cytotoxic T cells accounts for the accelerated rejection.

We have come a long way since Mary Shelley created Dr. Frankenstein, who created the Creature. If Mrs. Shelley were writing today she would have to include descriptive passages of how Dr. Frankenstein matched his collection of "parts" for MHC compatability and then gave cyclosporine and other immunosuppressive drugs to forestall the host-versus-graft rejection. The keeping of a new heart (or other organ) in place is still a tenuous affair, but scientists are gradually illuminating the immunological secrets of the Golem. The laborers in immune fields predict that the day is not far off when tissue transplantation can be accomplished with a surety equal to a "lifetime guarantee."

# Chapter 8

# Immunity au Naturel

THE LAST two chapters revealed the immune system to be remarkably effective, diverse, and responsive in dealing with pathogens and other substances recognized as foreign. The problem is that even the rapid secondary immune reactions enacted by memory B and T cells take time, and time can be a precious commodity in dealing with virulent microorganisms. It is a problem that confronts us from the very moment of birth. We are born sterile; in a state of microbial innocence we slide down the birth canal into a world teeming with both benign and pathogenic microbes. At this first moment of independent life we are threatened by overwhelming infection. Later in life we are at risk while waiting for the "immunological doctor" to arrive (an archaic metaphor if there ever was one), for the immune system to get its act together.

That we are not overwhelmed is due to nature—divine providence having endowed us with a nonspecific, first-line defense system that "instinctively" recognizes the hostile foreigners and is constantly at work in the control of infection. The components of this natural defense system are soluble factors in body fluids and specialized "policeman" cells.

## *The Good Humors of Natural Immunity*

During the early years of the twentieth century, immunological research was preoccupied with unraveling the mysteries surrounding the nature and origin of specific antibodies. The first line of defense, the natural immunity such as that attributed to the phagocytes by Metchnikoff, was largely ignored as a topic for major inquiry. Then sometime in 1921 or 1922, Sir Alexander Fleming had a drippy nose cold and by technical misadventure discovered an entirely new dimension of natural immunity (later, another technical misadventure led to Fleming's discovery of penicillin). Fleming was examining a petri dish in which colonies of bacteria were growing on nutrient agar when, in a moment of fixed concentration on his observations, a drop of mucus fell from his runny nose onto the agar. Most modern bacteriologists working with finicky precision in a sterile environment (a) would never have been so technically sloppy and, (b) if they had so grossly contaminated a culture plate would have consigned it directly to the waste bag. This was not Sir Alexander's technical style and he returned the petri dish to the incubator. When he examined the dish a few days later he saw to his surprise that the bacterial colonies had either disappeared or were very much reduced in size. Something in the mucus was destroying the bacteria. There was a "remarkable bacteriolytic element" in mucus, as Fleming noted in a paper published in 1922.

This element, which came to be named *lysozyme*, was later found to be present not only in mucus but also in tears, saliva, and within phagocytes. It also seems to be a primitive, "Garden of Eden" type of natural immune defense that arose early in evolutionary history since it is present throughout the animal kingdom, in invertebrates as well as in vertebrates.

Lysozyme is an enzyme that attacks the complex amino acid–sugar polymer which forms the outer cell wall of many bacteria. It causes the chemical dissolution of that wall in a manner akin to the meat tenderizer enzyme, papain, breaking down the protein molecule. Lysozyme is considered to be important in preventing infections of the mouth (including tooth decay) and eye. There is a rare, inherited condition, Sjögren's syndrome, in which lysozyme is either absent or at very low concentration in the saliva and tears. Those with this genetic abnormality are plagued with recurrent infections of the mouth and eyes.

Lactoferrin is another good humor of natural immunity. It is an iron-binding protein first described from milk but subsequently identified in saliva, bronchial mucus, tears, urine, cervical secretion, seminal fluid, and within phagocytic white blood cells. Transferrin, an iron-avid protein in the serum, is related to lactoferrin although it has a somewhat different chemical structure. Lactoferrin and probably transferrin are thought to suppress the growth of a number of microbial pathogens by out-competing them for available dietary iron, an element essential in their biochemical physiology.[1] There is a kind of "nutritional immunity" in having a mild iron-deficiency anemia (a severe anemia, on the other hand, depresses the immune system's responses). There are several examples where redressing the anemia has had unexpected untoward results. In one such unhappy incident drought-starved Somalis who were

1. Both microbes and host cells require iron to survive. It is not certain what the strategy is that allows the body to withhold iron from the microbe and provide it to its own cells. There is some evidence that the body can extract the iron bound to lactoferrin / transferrin, whereas the microbe lacks this mechanism.

hospitalized and abruptly shifted from a famine diet to nutritionally adequate hospital fare relapsed with clinically severe infections of malaria, tuberculosis, and brucellosis (Malta or undulant fever). The explanation offered: in their former iron-deficient state (the available iron being bound to lactoferrin / transferrin) the proliferation of these pathogens, which these people were infected with before coming to the hospital, was inhibited, thus imposing a state of clinical silence.

Another story of anemic success involves the Masai and the Zulus of Africa. Both tribes live, for the most part, under unhygenic conditions which would put them at high risk to becoming infected with *Entamoeba histolytica,* the cause of amoebic dysentery. However, clinicians had long noted that the Masai hardly, if ever, came down with amoebic dysentery while for the Zulu it was one of the most important of their health problems. The explanation that has been proposed to account for this difference is that the Masai, cattle herders, live almost exclusively on a cow's milk diet. Cow's milk has a very low iron content and most of what is present is bound to the lactoferrin. Amoebae need iron to live but they can't extract the iron from the lactoferrin. Anemic amoebae can't establish themselves in the Masai gut in numbers that would cause disease. The Masai, unlike the amoeba, can use what iron there is in milk although the low concentration makes him slightly anemic—but not so anemic that he can't kill a lion in hand-to-claw combat. Slight anemia is a good trade-off for freedom from gut- and liver-destroying amoebae. In contrast, the Zulu, who are omniverous, not only have a diet that is high in iron content but also cook their food in iron pots. During cooking, iron leaches from the pot to add still more metal to the meal. This excess of iron allows the amoebae to flourish.

Most of us are a long way from the Masai and Zulu. Coming closer to home it has been repeatedly proven that infants given the breast have significantly fewer intestinal infections (gastroenteritis) than infants who are formula-fed. This protection is afforded not only by the specific IgA antibodies in the milk that are bathing the baby's gut but also by the nonspecific, natural protective factors lactoferrin and another substance, lactoperoxidase.

Lactoperoxidase is still another natural antimicrobial humor in saliva, milk, and tears. Lactoperoxidase is an enzyme. It participates (catalyzes) a chemical reaction involving sugars, sulfur-containing compounds (thiocyanates), and hydrogen peroxide that ends in the production of end products that are bacteriostatic—they prevent the bacteria from multiplying.

Lactoperoxidase is considered to be particularly important in controlling bacterial overgrowth in the mouth. These bacteria flourish because we eat carbohydrate foods to supply them with the sugar fuel. It is this fuel that gives them the sexual (asexual really; bacteria don't have sex) energy they need for rapid replication. The sugar-metabolizing bacteria give off hydrogen peroxide. When the hydrogen peroxide reaches a critical concentration, the lactoperoxidase in the sugar goes to work to convert it to a bacteriostatic substance and in this way inhibits too florid a bacterial growth. Unfortunately, there is just so much lactoperoxidase and the constant intake of high-sugar-content foods will keep the bacteria multiplying.

## The Phagocytes on the Scrimmage Line

As you well know, one rarely leaves the doctor's office without tithing some blood for the diagnostic cause. The contribution is well worth the slight discomfort because blood constituents mirror, in myriad ways, the state of health and the specific abnormalities associated with an illness. The complete blood count (CBC) is the basic hematological workup and is usually the first set of values looked at. If you are a normal, healthy adult your CBC lab report would read something like the following list (don't worry if you're not right on the numbers; there is considerable range in normal values between individuals as well as differences due to age and sex):

| Hemoglobin | 15 grams / 100 ml blood |
|---|---|
| Hematocrit | 42% |
| (volume of packed red cells) | |
| Red blood cells | 5 million / cubic millimeter |
| White blood cells | 7,000 / cubic millimeter |

DIFFERENTIAL WHITE BLOOD CELL COUNT

| Neutrophils | 68% |
|---|---|
| Eosinophils | 1.5% |
| Basophils | 0.5% |
| Lymphocytes | 25% |
| Monocytes | 5% |

The red cell count, hemoglobin level, and hematocrit would indicate whether there is an anemia. The white cell count and its composition (differential count) give clues to other disorders. A rise in white cell numbers, particularly an increase in neutrophils, often betokens a bacterial infection. An increase in eosinophils is a common sign of infection with a parasitic worm or an allergic disorder. The neutrophils, eosinophils, and basophils are collectively known as polymorphonuclear granulocytes because their nucleus is segmented into lobes and they have granule-like inclusions within their cytoplasm. They are phagocytic cells. Furthermore, they are phagocytic cells that can go about their work without prior "instruction" from a microbial or other antigen. They are "professional" phagocytic cells and the neutrophil is the most professional of the professional killers. The augmentation of neutrophil numbers in the blood and their accumulation at the infected site represents the scrimmage line of immune defense.

Normally, there may "only" be approximately five thousand neutrophils in each cubic millimeter of blood but there are enormous reserves of these cells in the bone marrow, spleen, and adherent to the lining walls of blood vessels. While it may take days or weeks for antibody and T cell–mediated immunity to attain effective levels, the neutrophils can be called forth from the reserve pools within minutes or hours of microbial invasion.[2]

If neutrophils are all that good and quick at gobbling up microorganisms, then why would other kinds of immunity—antibody, T cells, other forms of phagocytes—ever be needed? The chief defect of the neutrophil as the Compleat Defender is its brief life span. It dies two or three days after leaving the bone marrow where it is birthed from rapidly dividing precursor cells. Another limitation is that it is a "kamikaze" phagocyte. After ingesting it, the neutrophil must attend to the essential business of actually killing the microbe. The neutrophil comes from the bone marrow production line with its metabolic battery at "full charge," a sizeable store of sugar that can be used for a quick conversion into energy. A series of enzymatic, energy-depen-

2. The signals that call forth the neutrophils from reserve to active status haven't been fully elucidated. Adrenalin and factors of the activated complement system are two signals that have been identified.

dent transactions takes place to effect this conversion and, in a metabolic sense, cremates the microbe. Unfortunately, it is a suicidal transaction that not only kills the microbe but the neutrophil also.

So, although neutrophils are marvelously efficient phagocytes, their short life span and tendency to self-destruct limit their usefulness to quick skirmishes on natural immunity's front line. However provident nature has provided a backup phagocyte for the longer term. This is the monocyte, a lymphocyte-like cell with a single, round nucleus. The monocytes attack microbes with less eagerness than do neutrophils and kill them, once ingested (phagocytized), rather more slowly. The monocyte's grace is that it is the durable, long-lived workhorse of natural immunity. It does not self-destruct. It continues to mop up and digest microbes and other particulate antigens after the neutrophils have been exhausted. The monocyte not only phagocytizes, it is also important as a cell that manufactures and secretes factors involved in immune defense. One such factor is a substance that induces a lymphocyte to mature into a T or B cell. Another factor secreted by the monocyte is lysozyme.

## Assassins for Immunity: The Natural Killer Cells

In progressing from the description of the "professional killer" phagocytic cells to that of another family of Assassins, the *natural killer (NK) cells,* the reader might mistake this for a discourse on criminal psychopathology. A white blood cell that looked like a lymphocyte except that it was somewhat larger and contained blue-staining granules was described in 1910. Not much was known about the functions of any of the white blood cells at that time other than the monocytes were phagocytic. It wasn't until the mid-

1970s that this odd-looking lymphocyte was shown to be a cytotoxic killer cell—a cell that kills its target not by phagocytosis but with secreted chemical destructors.

T cells (lymphocytes) that have a cytotoxic function were described in the preceding chapter. These cytotoxic T cells respond by coming into proximity to its specific target, such as the cells of a tissue graft, and giving it a chemical kiss of death. The cytotoxic T cells, like the other members of the T cell family, are preprogrammed. They respond to a specific antigen. You will recall that the dogma of immunological clonal selection proclaims that for every possible antigen / epitope there lies in waiting a specific lymphocyte. Upon presentation of that antigen the lymphocyte rapidly and repeatedly divides to become a population—an expanded clone—of reactive, mature T or B cells. In contrast, the "other" odd-looking lymphocytes that were larger and granular were found to conduct their affairs in a very different manner. They were more like the neutrophil professional killers in that they required no preliminary sensitization with consequent maturation and clone expansion. These lymphocytes went directly to a foreign target cell, adhered to it, and killed it by lysis (in a manner akin to the cytotoxic T cell)—hence the name "natural killer cells."

What made the natural killer cells of particular interest to immunologists was their primary targets—cancer cells, especially the cancer cells of blood-borne metastases. A number of cancer experts had despairingly philosophized that humans were supinely defenseless against cancer(s). Their argument ran that malignancies, as bad as they are, do not occur so frequently as to be a threat to the survival of the species. Ergo, the Darwinian view would hold that anticancer mutations would not be selected for as they arose and we and our mammalian relatives would not have evolved anticancer defenses. The debut of the natural killer cells largely changed this notion. It is now felt that evolution has supplied us with surveillance policemen led by the natural killer cells and although they obviously do not give us the guarantee of *absolute* protection, the body is not, in fact, supinely defenseless against cancer.[3] Moreover, this protective system may have been set in place when the evolutionary tree was still a sapling. The earthworm has cells that look similar to the natural killer cells and seem to have similar functions (with earthworms it is all natural immunity; they don't have acquired immune responses such as antibody formation).

The natural killer cells also recognize and destroy virus-infected cells and cells from donor tissues, particularly the cells of bone marrow transplants. Recent research suggests that the natural killer cells are programmed to "sense" all cells that are dividing at an abnormally rapid rate. It is not only cancer cells that proliferate rapidly but other tissue cells, such as intestinal epithelial cells and bone marrow cells, have a rapid rate of division and unless controlled may overgrow. Some workers now think that the natural killer cells play a regulatory role in preventing such an overgrowth.

---

3. Fifteen years ago, cancer researchers and immunologists were of the opinion that cancers were a normal part of life—that cancer cells arise in everyone each day of their life. It was postulated that a vigorous immune surveillance system, manned by natural killer cells, cytotoxic T cells, and macrophages, did away with the tumor cells before they could become established. Cancer occurred on those relatively rare occasions when they evaded the immune surveillance system. One current view is that cancer cells arise very infrequently, perhaps only once in a lifetime, and that the immune surveillance system is not as efficient as was formerly thought. Immune surveillance led by the natural killer cells is now thought to have its greatest effect against virus-induced cancers.

It should be pointed out that this is all very new; there is still much to be learned about these natural killers and how they work. It now seems that there is not one type of natural killer lymphocyte but a whole tribe of them that do different things in somewhat different ways. One of the tribe is called the *anomalous killer cell*—a name that has a ring of intrigue to it. Among the immunological fraternity there are those who remain doubtful of the natural killer cell's role in surveillance of cancer and other abnormal cells. In a recent critical review the immunologist-authors, Drs. Thomas Hoffman and Manlio Ferrarini, posed the question "Is natural killer activity an immunologist's toy?" After sifting through all the available evidence they came to the conclusion that the natural killer cell is not an artifact of "test-tube" experiment—it is the Real Thing.

## Complement: Immunity of the Third Kind

Humoral immunity, the elaboration of specific antibody, is one arm of the immune system. Cell-mediated immunity effected by cytotoxic lymphocytes (T cells and natural killer cells) and phagocytes is the second immune arm (of course, there is considerable interaction and cooperation between the two arms). The complement system, a hideously complex group of naturally occurring proteins in the serum, is the third arm of the immune system. Complement has a semispecific action in that it makes certain antibody reactions, notably the lysis of antigen targets, "go." It also has, by itself, a number of defensive properties of natural immunity.

In the closing decade of the nineteenth century the observation was made that when serum containing specific antibody against a bacteria was heated to 56°C for thirty minutes the antibody lost its ability to kill the bacteria by lysis. In the "test tubes" in which these experiments were carried out, the heat-inactivated serum would still clump the bacteria in specific fashion; it just wouldn't kill them. In follow-up experiments it was shown that only the antibody's lytic activity was inactivated and that the antibody itself was by no means destroyed by the heating. In those experiments an experimental animal was infected with the bacteria. Later the heat-inactivated, antibody-containing serum was inoculated into the animal. The bacteria were killed by the transferred antibody and the animal was cured. It was all very confusing.

In 1895, the Belgian Jules Bordet began to furnish the first explanations to account for these baffling observations. Bordet showed that if a small amount of fresh, unheated serum from a "clean," unimmunized animal was added to the heat inactivated, antibody-containing serum, then the lytic (bacteriolytic) potency was restored. Clearly, there was a substance in normal serum that could be destroyed by heating, and which acted in conjunction with antibody and was necessary for antibody to exert its lytic effect. Bordet called this factor "alexin." A few years later Ehrlich renamed it *complement,* and complement it has been ever since.

Bordet, Ehrlich, and my immunology professor in 1948 considered complement to be a single, soluble substance. It is now known that complement is a system consisting of nine major components and eleven subcomponents. All these components are proteins which together constitute about 5 to 10 percent of the total serum protein.

During the good times of health, the complement components circulate in the serum in an inactive, quiescent state. The complement system becomes energized in the course of an infection (and in certain other disease states). The process is like a chain reaction with one component energizing the next until the final, ninth component, becomes activated. Usually (in the "*classical pathway*," in immunological parlance) "ignition" takes place with the ménage à trois union of IgG or IgM molecule,[4] its destined antigen / epitope, and a molecule of the first component of the complement system. The final fall of the tumbler is the conversion of the ninth component, a series of conversions that are enzymatic and nonenzymatic events. The activated ninth component binds (in our example) to the bacteria's cell wall and dissolves a small portion, making a minute lesion. After numerous complement "hits," the bacterium's cell wall, when viewed under an electron microscope, looks like a piece of Swiss cheese. In this punctured condition the bacterium's vital juices, the cytoplasm, streams out (lysis) and the microbe dies. Thus, the complement system, a collection of interrelated natural humors, amplifies the service of antibodies.

Complement activation may also be induced directly, without participation of the IgG or IgM antibody molecules, by certain substances such as the chemicals composing bacterial cell walls, cell-membrane fragments, and DNA. This pathway, which is a form of natural immunity because it doesn't involve specific antibody, is called the *alternate pathway*. Ignition of the alternate pathway begins with activation of the fourth component in the sequence which

4. Of the five immunoglobulin classes only IgG and IgM can bind complement. They can do so because they have a specific receptor specific for the first component of complement on their Fc region (the stem portion of the Y immunoglobulin molecule). IgA, IgD, and IgE do not have a complement-binding receptor.

complementologists have labeled, to confound the unwary, component 3 (C3).

In both the classical and alternate pathways each activated component and subcomponent has certain biological activities. In the activation process certain fragments of complement are produced which also have biological activity. It is more than my editor or common sense would allow to go through this maze of activation. We make medical and graduate students recite the Complement Catechism and if they fail the test we pass them on to the secular arm. The reader who may himself or herself be "turned on" by complement should consult a recent textbook on immunology. And the best of luck to you. Anyway, here are some of the things that the activated components, subcomponents, and complement fragments do:

1. Kill viruses and other microbial pathogens directly (no antibody involved).

2. Stimulate macrophages to ingest microbes.

3. Cause the small blood vessels to dilate and become more permeable so that phagocytes and other cells of the immune system can more readily squeeze through the vessel walls and travel to the tissue areas where they are needed.

The importance of the natural immunity conferred by the complement system is evidenced by the disorders in those individuals with inherited defects in which one or more complement components are either absent or at an abnormally low concentration. Amongst other problems, these people suffer from recurrent bacterial infections, hereditary angioedema (attacks of swelling of the mucous membranes and skin eruptions from overly "leaky" blood vessels), and, probably, systemic lupus erythematosus.

These last three chapters have told of an impressive network of protective immunity—a primary physical barrier (the intact skin and mucous membranes), a second defensive line of natural humoral and cellular elements (including the complement system), and a formidable third line of defense, the specific humoral (antibody) and cell-mediated immune responses. But if the immune network is so impressive then why do we still have to take an antibiotic or drug to cure an infection? And why should we come down with an infection in the first place? Why can't "nature" always be relied upon to do the job? Well, the fact is that nature does do the job impressively well when we consider that without our natural and acquired (specific responses) immune defense, each scratch could lead to a lethal sepsis, and each of what we now call minor infections would be a life-threatening experience. However, there are pathogens (and I include tumor cells among them)—clever little buggers that they are—that have, through evolutionary selection, acquired strategies to evade the immune system's best shots. Some microbes and parasites have even had the effrontery to develop the means to live exclusively within macrophages—the very cells of the immune system that are supposed to do them in. Other pathogens antigenically disguise themselves as their host. They have surface receptors that can take host antigens, such as a serum protein, onto their surface, or manufacture host-like antigens. With this mimicry when the antibody molecule, or cytotoxic T cell, or phagocyte, comes looking for them, these pathogens say, in effect, "There ain't nobody here but us humans." Other microbes have developed a genetic machinery that can mutate so rapidly as to produce one different antigen after another. They change their antigenic character so frequently that the immune defense can't keep the pace. Other pathogens outwit the immune defenses by means that are still unfathomed. It is these pathogens that slip through the immune network that require the best shots of the pharmaceutical industry. But even for these "smart" pathogens the "immunological doctor" is on the way (its coming is foretold in the final chapter, "Promises, Promises").

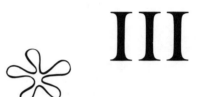

# III

## The Immune System in Sickness and in Health

# Chapter 9

# Eating Your Way
# to Immunity

IN A WORLD in which a quarter (or more) of humanity is malnourished it is cruelly paradoxical that diet has become a burning issue for the overnourished. The remedies for nuclear war, social injustice, and economic disarray all take second place to the tonnage of nostrums and advice we get for the care and feeding of the inner person. Of course, there are no pills or preparations against nuclear war or social injustice so these problems have no market value. But diet pills, preparations, and how-to books galore are available over the counter. Eating your way to health and perpetual youth is big business, with claims and counterclaims made by numerous factional partisans. However, this is a book about immunity, not nutrition, and I have no wish to enter into these larger dietary debates. It is sufficient to note that from every indication the immune system functions normally in those who enjoy a "normal" level of nutrition, that is, what is judged to be an adequate intake of calories and protein. The malnourished poor have a compromised immune response; I will deal with the nutritional indigent in a special section later in the chapter.

The chapter is primarily addressed to the "normals" whose immune system works well but who would like to evaluate strategies to make the immune system work bet-

ter than normal: to make it even more responsive in dealing with infection; to maintain a more youthful immune
system in the course of aging; and to increase the efficiency
of the natural killer and other specialized cells' patrols against
cancerous transformations.[1] Experimental research has
indicated that the way to a superefficient immune system
is by the supplementary intake of certain trace elements
and vitamins. I use the term "experimental" in a cautionary
sense. Nutritional research, including research on the dietary enhancement of the immune response, has been very
good research for the most part. The studies have been
tidy, often elegant and well controlled—and mostly of mice,
guinea pigs, and other experimental animals. Rarely have
humans been studied under the same controlled conditions
nor, in most cases, could they ethically be subjected to the
dietary manipulations imposed on experimental animals.
Immunonutritional studies on large population groups (epi-
demiological-type studies) and experimental studies on
humans with dietary deficiencies of disease-like proportions have helped provide a degree of insight and to confirm or refute some of the results from animals, but for the
most part our knowledge derives from research on experimental animals. Our human reader must decide, then,
whether the experimental evidence is sufficiently convincing and whether he or she is constitutionally similar enough
to a rodent to invest that five dollars for a bottle of selenium
or zinc or vitamin C—and to faithfully take the supplement
at a dosage that usually hasn't been fully proven to be effective in humans. With that caveat I'll begin with *my* favorite

1. As I noted in Chapter 8's discussion on natural killer cells, it is still a
bit iffy as to whether immune surveillance actually occurs in the body as
it does in the "test tube." I think that there is enough evidence for it to
merit our nutritional support.

immune-enhancer, selenium, a trace element that I've decided that if it's good enough for the mouse it's good enough for me.

## Selenium

I had used a selenium preparation, off and on, as an antidandruff shampoo for some years but what turned my head to its immunological potential was an article published by J. Spallholz in *Infection and Immunity* that promoted selenium, in minute amounts, as a phenomenal immune-enhancer in mice. Mice that had been given a selenium-supplemented diet raised a very much higher level of antibody after injection with an antigen (Spallholz used sheep red blood cells as the antigen in his experiments) than their similarly injected brethren mice fed an ordinary diet.

About that time I and one of my graduate students, John Barnwell, were having our own immunological problems. We had been trying to immunize mice against a rodent malaria, *Plasmodium berghei*, using various preparations of the parasite as vaccines. It was a "screening" project to give some indication of what might be an effective vaccine for humans against *their* malarias. Nothing worked. All the vaccinated mice died of a fulminating infection following challenge with live, virulent malaria parasites. Either there was something wrong with our vaccine antigens or there was something intrinsically defective in the mouse's immune system that didn't allow the development of a protective response. Spallholz's paper came to my attention and, as much in desperation as curiosity, we decided to try selenium as a booster of the mouse's immune response to our vaccines. We added two parts selenium per million parts of the their drinking water and, after two weeks on the selenium-ade, they were injected with a vaccine that had been prepared from an extract of the parasites. Two weeks after vaccination, they were challenged with an inoculation of living parasites. Not only did all the mice that had been given the selenium-supplemented drinking water live, but only a few parasites appeared in their blood for a brief period. They had become immunized. In contrast, the control mice that drank of the common tap water (and had been similarly vaccinated) all died of the typical unrelenting infection. Also about that time our research funding expired. I went on to other studies and (now Dr.) Barnwell went on to a postdoctoral fellowship, so we never undertook the next echelon of (very expensive) monkey-malaria experiments. Nevertheless, selenium had piqued my interest and I've tried to follow its progress in the biomedical literature. It would seem that this trace element can do a lot more than cure dandruff.

The need for *dietary* selenium was demonstrated approximately thirty years ago when it was observed that laboratory rats fed solely on torula yeast (which is selenium deficient) developed a kind of liver rot and died. Then it was discovered that domestic animals—chickens, calves, and lambs—became afflicted with a muscular disease, which included degeneration of the heart muscles, if they did not get enough selenium in their food and forage. The human linkup came in 1979 when medical scientists in the People's Republic of China described a fatal, degenerative disease of the heart, mostly affecting children, in Keshan Province. In Keshan the soil is almost devoid of selenium and, therefore, the plant and animal food has an abnormally low selenium content. Working on the animal analogy, the Chinese doctors gave sodium selenite to those with

Keshan's disease, as it came to be called. A dramatic, rapid improvement followed for those treated in this way.

Keshan's disease and the related diseases of domestic animals are abnormalities caused by a dietary intake *deficient* in selenium. Conversely, *too much selenium can be toxic*. Those of us (the great majority) on an adequate level of nourishment and dietary variety obtain a sufficient amount of selenium to satisfy our physiological requirements. That amount has been estimated by the National Research Council to be between 50 to 200 micrograms daily (a microgram, abbreviated as "mcg" on the store-bought bottle, is one-millionth of a gram). The new experimental studies indicate that if we take a *little bit more* than the physiological demand, the immune system becomes supereffective in a number of ways. The trick is not to take too much selenium—then selenium has the opposite effect, it becomes immunosuppressive *and may even be toxic*. The "just-right" immune augmentation dose for humans hasn't been fully worked out. In rats, it's about 10 micrograms selenium per kilogram body weight, daily (a 200-gram rat would be given 2 micrograms selenium daily). I hedge my own life's bets and take one drug-store-bought selenium pill of 200 micrograms every other day.

I noted earlier that the just-a-little-bit-more amount of selenium has a powerful effect in increasing antibody synthesis in experimental animals. Selenium has other notable effects on the immune system. First, it has an anti-inflammatory[2] effect. What is interesting is that experimen-

2. Inflammation has been defined as the "reaction of living tissue to injury, which comprises the series of changes of the terminal vascular bed, of the blood, and of the connective tissues that tends to eliminate the injurious agent and to repair the damaged tissue" (H. Z. Movat, in *Inflammation, Immunity, and Hypersensitivity*, [New York: Harper & Row, 1979]). This is the immune reaction characterized by the migration of

tally, vitamin E (DL-alpha tocopherol) greatly augments selenium's anti-inflammatory action although vitamin E *by itself* (except at very high doses) had little or no anti-inflammatory effect. The optimal dosage of a selenium–vitamin E combination for humans is not known. In rats, it was 12.5 milligrams (mg) vitamin E plus 10 micrograms (mcg) per kilogram body weight / selenium selenite. Unfortunately, drug dosages cannot always be calculated by the simple multiplication of rat-to-human body-weight ratios.

Undoubtedly the most intriguing and potentially important attribute of selenium is its attributed ability to prevent cancer. This is not a new concept. In what now seems like the medieval days of science in 1912, a French physician, P. Dalbert, wrote a paper advocating selenium as a treatment for cancer. However, there was a gap of thirty-seven years before Dalbert's hypothesis was put to the experimental test. From 1949 onwards numerous studies have been carried out on the value of selenium in preventing experimental cancers in rats and mice. Synoptically, these studies have proved that selenium prevented the occurrence in 50 to 100 percent of the skin, mammary, colon, and liver cancers that can be experimentally induced in those animals by carcinogenic chemicals and certain (oncogenic) viruses. Cancer was prevented when these experimental animals were given drinking water supplemented with two

phagocytes and other white blood cells to the injured or infected site. The inflammatory response is felt as localized heat and soreness.

There is also a group of "inflammatory diseases" in which the immune response does not lead to healing but to further tissue destruction. This is a diverse, poorly understood group of diseases which include skin conditions such as cutaneous necrotizing anginitis, and granulomatous diseases such as ulcerative colitis and Crohn's disease of the intestinal tract. A variety of drugs and biological agents (such as steroids) are used in an attempt to "cool down" these abnormal, hyperinflammatory conditions.

to six parts selenium per million parts (weight / volume) water. Both inorganic selenium in the form of sodium selenite and organic selenium from selenium-rich yeast[3] acted as cancer prophylactics, although the inorganic form has been reported to have a somewhat higher activity.

Experimentally, selenium has shown good value as a cancer preventitive; but will it cure if that microgram of prevention isn't there? The recent report (1984) by A. M. Watrach and his colleagues at the University of Illinois suggests that not only will selenium cure but that it can do so against cancer cells of human origin. These workers took cancer cells originating from a human breast tumor perpetuated in tissue culture, and inoculated the cells into mice. In the mice, the inoculated cells not only lived but grew into a cancerous mass. Some of these tumorous mice were then inoculated three times a week with .8 microgram sodium selenite per gram of body weight. After forty weeks the untreated mice were dying from the massive tumerous growth. In the selenium-treated mice there was a tumor, but it was minute in size—93 percent less in volume than the average size in the control animals. Watrach et al. had no theories as to how the selenium worked nor did they make any claim as to its relevance in the treatment of human cancer patients. But theirs is an intriguing, and possibly important, observation. Let us hope that this line of research will be pursued further.

There is no certainty that the causes of, and cures for, cancers of the rodent are the same for humans—although

3. There are two sodium salts of selenium, sodium selenite and sodium selenate. Sodium selenate is less toxic than the selenite but its activity in immunological and cancer studies has not been adequately assessed. The organic form of selenium is prepared from a variety of selenium-rich plants, most commonly from yeast. In Finland the organic selenium pill is made from the ashes of the birch tree.

there are enough similarities to keep a host of "mouse workers" busy and in funding dollars. Cancerwise, is selenium as beneficial for humans as it is for rats and mice? Since researchers would not (and could not) put a group of humans on a selenium-supplemented diet and then deliberately try to induce cancer with a carcinogen, oncogenic virus, or transplanted tumor cells, the answer to this question has had to come from epidemiologists—medical specialists who try to discern the factors contributing to health and disease under natural conditions. The epidemiologists dissected out the "selenium factor" by the following reasoning. People get their selenium from the plants they eat or by eating the meat of the animals which have eaten the plants. The plants get *their* selenium from the soil. The soil in different parts of the United States (and in different parts of the world) have different levels of selenium content. *Ergo*, if selenium prevents cancer, then there should be less cancer in areas with a high selenium content in the soil (and plant foods grown there) than in areas where the soil selenium is low.

Experimentalists, with their tidy cages of inbred mice, have a much better lot than epidemiologists, who must deal with the unruly masses. In examining for the effect of selenium, epidemiologists had to make all sorts of allowances for factors experimentalists can control. The epidemiologists had to manipulate their statistical analyses to take account of age and sex ("broken down by age and sex" as the epidemiological pun goes), factors which relate to the incidence of different kinds of cancer. Allowance had also to be made for any regional variations in dietary habits and food consumption. Interpretation of the data could also be confounded by differences in life-styles, such as urban versus rural. Despite these limitations, the studies carried out so far have indicated, after adjusting for the confounding factors, a statistically lower incidence of cancer in the high-selenium areas than in the low-selenium areas. In one of these investigations, two epidemiologists, R. J. Shamberger and C. E. Willis, who took as their "yardstick" the selenium in forage crops, reported lower numbers of deaths (mortality rates) due to cancers of the breast, lung, digestive tract, and lymphoid tissues in areas where the forage crops had a higher selenium content than in the areas where the plants had a low selenium content. Recently (1983), U. M. Cowgill reassessed all the data from studies carried out so far and came to the same conclusion—that there was less cancer, particularly of the lung, digestive organs, and breast, in the geographical areas where the forage crops have a high selenium content.

I don't advocate a mass exodus to the selenium-high states, although you might consider the prudence of taking a selenium supplement pill if you live in a low-selenium area. There are, also, differences in soil selenium levels from county to county within any one state. A table gives an overall guide to the states' selenium states. (Sorry, I have no data for Alaska or my home state, Hawaii.)

There is no Grand Unified Theory as to how selenium works in enhancing the immune system or in its anticancer properties. The best guesses are that selenium has several modes of action. One postulate holds that selenium super-charges the mitochondria of cells. Mitochondria are minute, sausage-shaped structures within all nucleated cells. They are the cell's dynamo, transforming fuel into energy. A highly energized cell of the immune system could, theoretically, lead to the production of a greater amount of antibody and to the more rapid proliferation of T and B

SOIL SELENIUM LEVELS IN THE
CONTINENTAL UNITED STATES

| HIGH | MEDIUM | LOW |
| --- | --- | --- |
| Alabama | California | Connecticut |
| Arizona | Georgia | Delaware |
| Arkansas | Idaho | District of Columbia |
| Colorado | Kentucky | Florida |
| Iowa | Minnesota | Illinois |
| Kansas | North Carolina | Indiana |
| Louisiana | Oregon | Maine |
| Mississippi | South Carolina | Maryland |
| Missouri | Tennessee | Massachusetts |
| Montana | Virginia | Michigan |
| Nebraska | Washington | New Hampshire |
| Nevada | | New Jersey |
| New Mexico | | New York |
| North Dakota | | Ohio |
| Oklahoma | | Pennsylvania |
| South Dakota | | Rhode Island |
| Texas | | Vermont |
| Utah | | West Virginia |
| Wyoming | | Wisconsin |

cells, the secretion of more lymphokines, and to phagocytes devouring foreign particulate antigens even more voraciously than they do normally.

Selenium also acts as an antioxidant and this may also have an important bearing on its immuno-enhancing and anticancer effects. The enzyme-mediated conversion of fuel—sugars, proteins, and particularly fats—into energy results in the production of superoxides as end-product "fallouts" of the bioenergetic train. Superoxides are oxygen and oxygen-containing substances whose oxygen atoms have one less electron than the normal oxygen atom. Hydrogen peroxide is one such superoxide that is a metabolic end product. There are environmental superoxides, in ever-increasing amounts, in the air we breath—ozone and nitrogen dioxide. Superoxides are toxic to the cell. They damage cell membranes and cripple the cell's power plant, the mitochondrion. There is an enzyme, glutathione peroxidase, which needs selenium to convert the poisonous superoxides to harmless alcohol (vitamin E, another antioxidant, acts by directly combining with, and inactivating, the superoxide). These antioxidants are thought to protect against cancers by a dual action, the enhancement of immune surveillance and by direct inactivation of tumor promoters. [4]

The antioxidant protection by selenium may become defective in sickness, malnutrition, and old age. This results in defective cell function. Impaired cell function results in poorer immunity and a generally poorer state of health.

Senescence is due, in part, to the metabolic flame burning the oils (lipids) less and less efficiently. With advanced age the glutathione peroxidase–selenium enzyme doesn't work as well as in the salad days of our youth and noxious

4. Agents that can cause cancer can be divided into two types of substances—carcinogens and tumor promoters. Carcinogens initiate the transformation of normal cells to the neoplastic state—they are direct cause of cancers. Certain coal-tar products, for example, are carcinogens. Tumor promoters by themselves do not cause cancers. The promoters may be no less important in the development of clinical cancer than the carcinogens. If an animal (presumably including the human animal) is exposed to a very small amount of the carcinogen no tumor will develop; there is a quantitative threshold of exposure necessary. However if that same small amount of carcinogen is given together with a promoter *then* a tumor will develop. So far only a few tumor promoters have been identified and these are mainly substances derived from fungi, algae, and higher plants. There is also evidence that certain parasitic worms may be tumor promoters. Epidemiological evidence suggests that the worldwide variation of cancer incidence may be due to the variation of human exposure to tumor-promoting substances.

oxidants accumulate. In a literal sense we may, as we age, be rusting out. There is a remarkable study from Finland that indicates that a combination of selenium and vitamin E may be "rust retardant." The study was carried out by a research team from the University of Helsinki on a group of residents, average age seventy-six years, in an old-age home. The "best of yet to be" had passed these people by; they were confused, depressed, anxious, unable to care for themselves, constantly fatigued, and had little appetite for food or life. One half of the group were given a daily dose of 8 milligrams of sodium selenate (remember! this is the *selenate*. The *selenite* would be toxic at this dosage) in two divided doses, 45 micrograms of organic selenium (a birch ash pill), and 400 milligrams of vitamin E. The other half of the group, the controls, were given "dummy" placebo pills. It was a double-blind experiment and neither the patients, pill-givers, nor those who assessed the results knew who got the selenium–vitamin E and who got the dummy pill. A quantitative test, the Sandoz Clinical Assessment Geriatric-scale, which measures the overt parameters of senescence, was applied to determine whether or not the treatment had any effect. Within two months those on the selenium–vitamin E showed a marked, statistically significant improvement (as compared to the control group). They became less depressed; they began to care for themselves; they were less fatigued and less hostile; they had more initiative and a renewed appetite. One patient felt so well that he left the home (and the experiment). However, the supplementation wasn't *absolutely* perfect and there was no improvement in memory. This is the kind of study that needs repeating for confirmation. I predict that selenium–vitamin E will become important as a therapy in geriatric care. My own expectation is that selenium and vitamin E—and the acquisition, by some miracle, of a forehand volley—will get me to Wimbledon's centre court by the time I'm sixty-five.

## Vitamin C (Ascorbic Acid)

The effect of vitamin C deficiency has been recognized since the late 1700s when Captain Cook gave limes to his sailors and thus prevented and cured scurvy. Today, most of us obtain sufficient vitamin C from what may euphemistically be called the "normal, balanced" diet. No one argues about the physiological necessity of including an adequate source of vitamin C in the diet. However, since March 1976, when Linus Pauling published his paper "Vitamin C and the Common Cold," the vitamin has been a center of controversy that extends far beyond its established antiscorbutic property. Today there are passionate advocates of the Mega C Faith, and debunkers who deny with equal intensity.

Pauling maintains that mammoth doses of vitamin C, a gram daily, reduces the illness caused by the common cold by approximately one-third. Considering the popularity and importance of the debate, there have been relatively few double-blind studies[5] to resolve the issue. In one double-blind study, carried out by I. M. Baird and his colleagues, it was concluded that vitamin C, even at doses as low as 80 milligrams daily, had a statistically significant effect in reducing the sickness caused by colds. Other studies,

5. Hope springs eternal in the heart of the researcher, hence the double-blind trial in which neither the physician-evaluator nor the patient-subject knows who received the treatment (such as a drug) and who the placebo (or other type of "dummy" control). At the termination of the trial, after the results are in and processed, a third party who has held the sealed code reveals who got what.

including those sponsored by the National Institutes of Health, came to the conclusion that vitamin C, at any dosage, does not protect against acquiring a cold or reduce the intensity or duration of the cold once it has been acquired. After scrutinizing all the evidence I have come to the opinion that vitamin C does have some action against the cold virus(es) but not as much as touted by its advocates. This is in agreement with B. Leibovitz and B. V. Siegal, who stated in their authoritative review, "These results taken together indicate a protective effect of ascorbic acid against the common cold; however it is unlikely that ascorbic acid is beneficial in all circumstances, and it should not be viewed as a panacea for such infections."

The fact that vitamin C at high doses (at least one-half gram daily) has been shown to have some value in other experimental and human viral infections such as mumps, herpes, measles, and influenza lends credence to its curative and preventive effect against the common cold. However, evidence is still lacking as to why and how vitamin C acts on this broad range of viruses. It does not act directly on the virus, like an antiviral drug, so it's more likely to exert its effect indirectly by stimulating the body's immunological defenses. A few pieces of information suggest that this may be the case. In one experiment, human volunteers were given 5 grams of vitamin C over a period of three days. At the end of this period, a blood sample was taken and the lymphocytes separated and tested for their ability to transform—to proliferate and mature—into functional T cells. After the vitamin C, the T cells were more activated—they showed a higher degree of transformation—than before taking the vitamin C regimen. In mice, vitamin C increases interferon production, the secretion of lymphocytes and other cells of the immune system that prevents viral invasion. There is also experimental evidence that the macrophages from vitamin C–treated mice have a higher level of microbicidal activity than nontreated "normal" mice. So there is some rationale for vitamin C therapy of the common cold. It's not a sovereign remedy but certainly is as good as, if not better than, chicken noodle soup.

## Vitamin A (Retinol)

Is it true what they say about vitamin A? The mouse men think so. E does it. C does it. And A may do it even better.

Similar to most of the other vitamins, A originally became best known for what it did as a deficiency rather than as an excess. Vitamin A, as all you night fighters out there know, is the stuff from which the light-sensitive pigment in the eye's retina is manufactured. Without adequate vitamin A intake there is less retinal pigment and this leads to a loss in visual acuity. A sustained deficiency can lead to blindness (lack of pigment, as will be noted in a moment, is only part of the cause of vitamin A deficiency blindness).

Some seventy years ago another, equally vital, activity of vitamin A came to light. The vitamin was found to be necessary for the controlled growth and integrity of epithelial cells. Epithelial cells are the cells that line the body's tracts and ducts; they form the surface of skin and membranes. They clothe the cornea and conjunctiva. Most epithelial cells are rapidly dividing cells that die and are replaced every few days. Vitamin A sees to it they don't divide *too* rapidly and that they remain as normal, functional epithelial cells. Without their mete of vitamin A, the epithelial cells become "horny"—keratinized. In the mucous membranes and respiratory tract, the "horny" cells stop secreting enough mucus and, it is conjectured, the natural antimicrobial lysozyme to maintain the natural protective barrier. This opens the way to infection; and, to quote a contemporary authority on the subject, "No nutritional deficiency is more completely synergistic with infection than vitamin A, as amply demonstrated both in laboratory animals and humans."[6] The keratinization of the epithelial cells causes the opacity of the cornea that contributes to blindness and chronic infections of the eye. And when the epithelial cells of the reproductive tract become vitamin A deficiency–horny, infertility follows.

We now come to the juncture where vitamin A may, potentially, most influence our lives. At this juncture there is cancer and its possible prevention. About fifty years ago, it was noted that cancers occurred with abnormally high frequency in people with vitamin A deficiency. When scientists came to ponder upon this, the relationship between vitamin A deficiency and cancer was perfectly logical. The cancers were of epithelial cell origin—the most common, lethal, and untreatable form of cancer. These are, for example, cancers of the lung, colon, and bladder. In experimental animals maintained on a diet devoid of vitamin A, their epithelial cells divided unrestrainedly, piled up one upon the other, and lost their characteristic structure. These were precancerous cells. In many of the experimental mice, they progressed to become cancers of the lung and intestine. It was reminiscent of the cellular transformations induced by carcinogens and their promotors.

Not long after the vitamin A deficiency–cancer association was made, investigations began on the converse effect.

6. Charlotte G. Neumann in *Malnutrition and the Immune Response*, ed. R. M. Suskind (New York: Raven Press, 1977), p. 364.

If the lack of vitamin A caused, or contributed to, cancer, then would an excess (an amount above the required minimum dietary intake) *prevent* cancer? A typical experiment would be one in which the skin of mice were painted with a hydrocarbon carcinogen (a benzene-like compound) followed by application of a tumor promoter such as croton oil. The mice would then be given a vitamin A supplement in their diet or a series of injections of the vitamin (or a synthetic analog of the vitamin). The carcinogen / promoter would first cause a wartlike growth (papilloma) which normally would undergo a second cellular tranformation to become a lethal skin cancer. In the mice given the vitamin A treatment, the papilloma would not develop into a cancer. The cells would die and the precancerous growth would disappear. Experiment after experiment over the past thirty or so years in mice, hamsters, guinea pigs, and rabbits have confirmed the power of vitamin A to prevent carcinogen- and virus-induced cancers of epithelial origin in the lung, intestinal tract, urinary tract, and other organs.

Two pertinent findings have emerged from all those experiments. (1) Derivatives and synthetic analogs have a greater prophylactic potency than vitamin A itself. At the moment, the synthetic, retinoic acid, seems to stand at the top of the prophylactic list. In mice, 25 to 300 micrograms of retinocic acid given daily seems to be the optimal dose range. (2) Vitamin A and its analogs, while able to prevent experimental cancers, cannot cure cancer, at any dosage, once the cancer has become established. There is, however, one intriguing study which showed that if animals with experimentally induced cancers were given vitamin A, then the X rays and drugs used to treat the cancer became more effective. There is also one study on humans with inoperable lung cancer that reported a slight, but measurable, retardation of the progress of their cancer after they had been given the vitamin A analog, retinyl palminate.

Research carried out during the past five years in such geographically separate laboratories as the Salk Institute in California and the Kyushu School of Medicine in Japan has given the first insights into how vitamin A operates as a cancer preventitive. The mechanism appears to be an immunological one. For reasons that are still not clear, vitamin A (and its analogs, of course) possesses the unique ability to stimulate cytotoxic, and only cytotoxic, killer T cells to recognize precancerous cells with greater sensitivity, proliferate more rapidly after they recognize the neoplastic cells, and kill the target abnormal cells with enhanced efficiency. These cytotoxic T cells are, you will recall, the cells of the immune system that are considered to be highly important in scavenging for abnormal, precancerous cells as they arise.

So should you take out the vitamin A cancer insurance? If I were a mouse I'd certainly take vitamin A. The difficulty as a human is that there has been very little in the way of human experimentation to confirm that it works in our species. And if it does work, at what dosage and in what chemical form? A diet rich in vitamin A would seem to be prudent and maybe a proprietary capsule wouldn't hurt. *But remember, don't take too much!* A large excess of vitamin A will turn you yellow. This may be one way of showing your solidarity with the Third World, but since an overdose is also toxic there are better ways to show your colors.

## Zinc

Zinc is one of those vague metals I know to be of great practical importance but I am not quite certain why. Batteries? Rustproofing? An ointment, zinc oxide, that my mother used to put on my cuts and sores—or was that the paint pigment? Even within this ambit of haziness, zinc as a dietary necessity, the kitchen zinc, is not well-registered in our individual or collective consciousness. As it turns out, eating your zinc is essential for your health and immune function.

Like many other dietary trace substances, such as vitamins, the medical importance of zinc was discovered in a negative, subtractive way through recognizing the syndrome of illness in people whose diet was chronically deficient in the element. The syndrome—poor growth, anemia, heightened susceptibility to infection, slow wound healing—was first described in the Middle East. In this region of the world the poor and semipoor have a diet that almost exclusively consists of cereals and unleavened bread. This highly fibrous diet is not only zinc-deficient but actually interferes with the absorption of what little zinc is in the food. When stunted Arab children were given zinc-rich meat or zinc pills they began to grow at a normal rate and the other abnormalities also began to abate. Then in 1973 K. M. Hambridge and his colleagues showed that many Western urchins weren't faring much better. This group reported that 37 percent of the children from American low-income families were below the height norm for their age and that their blood plasma had an abnormally low concentration of zinc. This was attributed to the low-meat, low-zinc diet that is the poverty-level cuisine. Moreover, about 10 percent of the children from affluent (at least middle-income) families, on their mono-diet of fibrous carbohydrate, such as pizza and donuts, weren't doing too well growth- and zincwise either.

Next, the experimentalists with their mice and special zinc-deficient diets began to make their contribution. Animal experimentation during this past decade has provided further insights into the human condition and has confirmed the immune system's multifaceted need for zinc. The most striking abnormality noted in experimental animals maintained on zinc-deficient diets was the rapid atrophy of the thymus gland. In Chapter 7, the thymus was described as the manufacturing center where T lymphocytes are finished into mature immunocompetent cells. It was also noted that, with age, the thymus becomes smaller until it has almost completely atrophied during our Golden Years. In old age, T cells become fewer and feebler in their immune activities. Mice fed a zinc-deficient diet were propelled into premature immunological senility. There was an accelerated reduction in the size of the thymus, and T cell functions became impaired. Cell-mediated immune responses such as lymphokine production and antibody production to T cell–dependent antigens all suffered from the lack of zinc. Also, phagocytes didn't devour bacteria and other particulate antigens with their customary voracity.

It is now well established that too little zinc in the diet is harmful to health. There is also an accumulating body of evidence that an extra amount, over and above nutritional needs, has an immunological booster effect somewhat like that of selenium. The results of the few studies that have been carried out along these lines are tantalizing and one could only wish that further research be encouraged. Two of the more intriguing investigations have shown that if too little zinc makes you immunologically old before your time then a "little more" zinc than normal might restore you, in old age, to immunological youth.

At the age of two a mouse is an ancient, comparable to an eighty-year-old human. The senile two-year-old mouse exhibits the same age-associated decline in immune function as do old humans. One of the ways to demonstrate this is to inject an old and a young mouse with the same antigen. After an appropriate period, the spleen of each animal is removed and processed to harvest a pure suspension of splenic lymphocytes (the spleen is packed with lymphocytes). The lymphocytes are placed in a culture fluid to which has been added the immunizing antigen. Under these culture (*in vitro*) experimental conditions the B cells (usually with the assistance of their friends the helper T cells) divide repeatedly, transform into plasma cells, and begin to secrete antibody into the culture fluid. Repeated studies of this kind show that lymphocytes from an old mouse produce much less antibody than the lymphocytes from a young mouse. In 1983, a collaborative group of researchers from Johns Hopkins University and the National Institute of Aging carried out a study of the design just described. What they also did was to add a minute amount of zinc chloride—a concentration of 1:10,000—to the culture medium containing lymphocytes from immunized young and old mice. The lymphocytes from the young mice responded to the zinc by elaborating 30 to 40 percent more antibody than the control lymphocytes from the same animal but cultured in a medium without the zinc additive. This is a remarkable stimulatory effect but even so, it's negligible when compared to zinc's action on the tired lymphocytes from old mice. Zinc enhanced the antibody production of these lymphocytes five- to twelve fold—500 to 1,200 percent! The lymphocytes had been restored to immunological youth in their ability to transform and manufacture antibody.

All well and good, but these rejuvenating events took place in a test tube, using lymphocytes from a two-year-old mouse. Would zinc have the same effect on the immune system of an eighty-year-old human? The first indication that the test tube does recapitulate real life has come from a group of Belgian researchers led by Dr. Jean Duchateau of the Saint Pierre University Hospital in Brussels. Duchateau gave a 220-milligram zinc sulfate pill, twice a day for a month, to a group of aged individuals all over seventy and with an average age of eighty-one. At the end of the one-month period, the group given the zinc were inoculated with tetanus vaccine along with an age- and sex-matched untreated control group. Later, when their immune systems had time to respond, blood was withdrawn and the level of antitetanus antibody measured. The group that had been given the zinc supplement produced a significantly greater amount of antibody than did the control group.

Normally, people of advanced age don't respond too well to vaccines. Antibody production is low and consequently immunization affords a poorer protection than in the young. If Duchateau et al. are right then the elderly might be better protected if they were prepared with a course of supplementary zinc before being given their immunizing shots. Duchateau's study also provided information as to the mechanism of zinc's restorative effect. The *total number* of lymphocytes didn't alter in the zinc-supplemented group of people. What changed was the proportion of the T cell–B cell ratio. There was a marked increase in the proportion of T cells in those given zinc and the T cells exhibited youthful immunological capacities and capabilities. This indicated a restoration of thymic function. Perhaps the Fountain of Youth is, at least in part, made of zinc.

"You should live so long," as my grandmother used to say, but demographic structure would have it that only a minority of this book's readers will be over eighty years old. Therefore, it's likely to be of more direct interest to you whether taking a zinc supplement would benefit the young middle aged and the old middle aged. Duchateau & Co. attempted to answer this also and, in a 1981 paper published in the *American Journal of Clinical Nutrition*, they recounted how they had given 660 milligrams of zinc sulfate (this is ten times the estimated dietary need) divided in three doses daily of 220 milligrams, for one month, to a group of young adults twenty to thirty years old. In this study, only T cell function was measured, an accepted correlate of the level of immune status and potential. After a month on the zinc, there was modest—but statistically significant—increase, 17 to 28 percent, in T cell responsive function. Again, this points to zinc's thymic activation. The question for the young and vigorous is whether it's worth taking a daily zinc supplement to obtain this degree of immunological increment. Probably not.

There have been two other revelations of zinc's golden power. In one study, zinc has been shown to accelerate wound healing while in the second study it has proved to be a cold remedy that outrivals vitamin C.

The healing of traumatic and surgical wounds is a complex process involving many cell lines, not least of which are the cells of the immune system. One group of investigators reasoned that a zinc-stimulated immune system would speed the healing of a surgical wound. The captive experimental "audience" to test this hypothesis was a group of healthy young U.S. Air Force servicemen. That is, they were healthy in all respects except that they required surgery to excise a pilonidal cyst, a congenital cyst of lower back or "tailbone" region which frequently becomes infected. Following surgery, one group was given a 220-milligram zinc sulfate capsule three times a day until the wound was completely healed. The control group, recovering from the same surgical procedure, was given the same postoperative care and medication but no zinc supplement. The two groups were then followed to determine if there would be a difference in repair rate. Zinc was a clear winner. The wounds of the patients given the zinc supplement were completely healed after forty days while those not given zinc took, as an average, eighty days for their wounds to heal.

This authoritative study was published in a prestigious medical journal in 1969. It obviously had great import on postsurgical patient care but suprisingly, as of this writing, no follow-up investigations have been carried out to confirm and extend the original observations. And certainly zinc supplementation has not become routine as a preoperative therapy. Why was this promising line not pursued? One possible reason (alibi really) is that it came in the midst of a twenty-year period—from 1960 to 1980—that witnessed some of biomedical science's most exciting discoveries, notably the cracking of the genetic code and the subsequent advances in genetic engineering and other aspects of molecular biology. Scientists and resources were directed to these glamorous enterprises (which have not necessarily led to an improvement of our life and health). Dietary studies, such as on the immunoregulatory effects of zinc, while never completely dropped, took second place despite the popular interest in relationships between nutrition and health. In fact, the popular interest may have tainted this area of research for the biomedical panjandrums. It was no longer "pure" science.

Zinc was turned to the common cold by a leukemic three-year-old girl from Austin, Texas, who didn't like to swallow pills. Maintaining an adequate level of nutrition is a particular problem during the prolonged combat with childhood leukemia. As we all know, one has to be well (or starving) to hunger for food. Vitamin and trace metal deficiencies can accompany eating like "a (sick) bird," compounding an already dire condition, a fact that too many physicians are not mindful of. Fortunately, this particular little girl's doctor was one of the mindful and as part of her dietary support he prescribed zinc gluconate pills. He was also aware of zinc's immuno-enhancing properties and hoped it might help correct the immunological defects and abnormalities characteristic of leukemia. There was, however, one almost insurmountable difficulty; this little girl adamantly refused to swallow pills. Persuading a three year old, especially a sick and crotchety three year old, requires the skill of a professional arbitrator-diplomat-parent. Finally, a compromise was reached; she wouldn't have to swallow the pill but she would suck on them, lozenge-fashion.

After she began taking zinc pills a remarkable change occurred—not to the status of the leukemia, but to her resistance to colds. The disease and the immunosuppressive therapy used to treat the disease had made her uncommonly susceptible to the common cold. There were few intervals in her young life when she was free of a cold's symptoms. Unexpectedly, after she began sucking zinc the colds were fewer, further between, and of much shorter duration when they did occur. In fact, her father noted that if she took the zinc lozenge at the *onset* of symptoms then the cold never bloomed and the symptoms disappeared within a few hours.

Both physician and parents were delighted by this therapeutic turn of clinical events. Most practitioners would be satisfied with the improvement of their patient but in this instance the father and doctor were sufficiently impressed to make them advocates of zinc versus the cold and they invested their energies and money in setting up a larger trial that might confirm zinc's anticold activity. They also enlisted the collaboration of a nutritional scientist from the University of Texas who assisted in evaluating the data and acted as a referee of a double-blind trial. They collected 146 volunteers who were given, as soon as they noticed typical cold symptoms, either an 180-milligram zinc gluconate pill (23-milligram zinc base) or a dummy look-alike pill that contained no zinc. Those conducting the trial didn't know who got the zinc and who got the dummy pill until all the results were in. The volunteers were told to suck on the pill for at least ten minutes so that the zinc (if it were a zinc pill) could bathe the throat epithelial tissues where the cold virus (rhinovirus) multiplies. When all the results were in and analyzed zinc was clearly confirmed as an anticold agent. Those taking the fake pill (placebo) endured their colds an average of 10.8 days while those faithfully sucking their daily zinc gluconate pill were completely cured in an average of 3.9 days. Some of those on zinc had their colds totally aborted after the initial symptoms. It was observed that for zinc to have its optimal effect it should be taken (only lozenge use is effective for the cold) as soon as possible after the first sniffle and other symptoms appear. This is the time when the virus is replicating within the host's cells.

During the writing of this discourse in praise of zinc, I

began to come down with my own cold and, putting my mouth where my pen was, I purchased a bottle of zinc gluconate pills from the local drug store and began to suck a pill a day despite its bitter taste. I wish to report that the cold died aborning. A few days of very mild sniffles that didn't even require resort to paper tissues—and that was it! It's anecdotal, and not good science, but I add my experience as one more statistic. And the little girl? Last report had it that she was cured of her leukemia although no claim is being made that zinc contributed to the cure.

How does zinc work? In the case of the cold it has been proposed that zinc, unlike vitamin C, has a direct killing effect on the replicating virus, which explains why sucking the pill to give direct contact between virus and zinc is more effective than swallowing the pill. In addition, zinc may also stimulate the immune response to bring about an early termination of the infection. In the other, preceding examples, zinc's immuno-enhancing activities has been explained by the mechanism of thymic rejuvenation. This line of reasoning would have it that zinc stimulates the production and action of the thymic hormones which regulate T cell maturation in the thymus. Thymic hormones and, consequently, cell-mediated immune responses are reduced in zinc-deficient animals. It is also known that zinc participates in the biochemical transformations wrought by at least one hundred enzymes. One of these zinc-dependent enzymes is thymidine kinase, which helps assemble the nucleotides—the building blocks—of the DNA needed for rapidly diving cells such as turned-on T lymphocytes.

Finally, knowing what we know today, when would one be advised to take supplementary zinc? If I were young and in my prime I wouldn't take it all the time. It's probably not needed for the normals under fifty years of age and may even be immunosuppressive for that group when taken continuously. I would seriously consider taking a daily supplementary pill of, 200 to 500 milligrams zinc gluconate or sulfate with the approach of my sixtieth or seventieth birthday. Zinc therapy should also be considered for the treatment of those pathological conditions in which there is a depression of T cell numbers and function. And, finally, when you feel a cold coming on give zinc a go!

## The Immunity of the Nutritionally Indigent

I OPENED this chapter by noting that 25 percent or more of humanity aren't getting enough to eat. This is a complex spectrum of undernourishment that grades from the marginally hungry to those starved to death. It is further complicated by other variables. Hunger can be seasonal: feast during the harvest season and famine during the dry months of fallow. Hunger can be behavioral. The cultural, ritualized impositions on food habits as often as not make no nutritional sense. Food taboos may deny nutriment in the midst of plenty to those who need it most, children and pregnant and lactating women. But most of all, hunger is caused by too many people and too little food.

In the Hungry (Third, Developing) World the trouble arises from the dual shortage of protein-rich food and overall food intake to meet energy requirements (the calories to burn and fuel the body machine) a condition known as *protein energy malnutrition (PEM)*. In its severest form, PEM leads to kwashiorkor and marasmus.[7] Then too, PEM is almost always compounded by vitamin and trace element deficiencies. Obviously, if you're too poor to buy food you won't have the wherewithal to buy the supplement pills to make up for the vitamins and trace metals that you aren't getting in the food you're too poor to buy.

There is no absolute agreement amongst nutritionists as to the minimal or optimal protein and caloric requirements. Those requirements are dependent on age, sex, height / weight, and level of customary activity. The World Health Organization / Food and Agriculture Organization joint expert committee have provided one comprehensive guideline of daily calorie-protein needs. For example, based on the committee's recommendations, a young to middle-aged (twenty to forty years old) 140-pound male who is not engaged in energetic work—a professor or author—would need 3,000 calories and 37 grams of good-quality protein per day. His female age-weight-activity counterpart could get along on 2,200 calories and 33 grams protein. If our model male was a hard-working farmer or laborer he would need about 4,000 calories and 50 grams of protein daily. Children, growing and active, need twice as many calories and grams of protein per kilogram body weight as does an adult. And pregnant women are indeed eating for two: they

7. Some authorities consider these two conditions to be the same, i.e., expression of severe PEM. Other authorities who are just as authoritative maintain that kwashiorkor results from insufficient protein even though enough food is eaten to meet energy / caloric requirements whereas marasmus results from deficient protein *and* caloric intake. Clinically, these authorities describe kwashiorkor as more acute in children under one year of age and marasmus as a more chronic condition of older children. In both conditions, one witnesses an apathetic child, stunted in growth. The body is wasted and bloated by edema. The skin is thin and depigmented. Untreated, these children die directly of PEM or killed by an infectious disease to which they are highly susceptible.

will need an extra 80,000 calories over the course of their pregnancy.

The minimal dietary quantities recommended by the expert committee are for their "reference" male or female: a clean, healthy, uninfected human. But the 25 percent of humanity that is hungry is not like the "reference" male or female. For one thing, *that* 25 percent is, for the most part, the same 25 percent of the world's population that harbors an intestinal zoo of parasitic worms. These worms not only divert food for their own use but also impede the absorption of nutriments, particularly amino acids, from the intestinal tract.[8] To add to this burden, the marginally nourished and undernourished of the Third World invariably live in absolutely apalling conditions. They lack a sewage system and clean water. As a result, from earliest childhood their life experience is of frequent, recurrent episodes of diarrhea. The constant reinfection with pathogenic intestinal bacteria and viruses leads to damage of the intestinal tract's lining and this, in turn, leads to defective absorption of nutriments from the gut. During the frequent acute episodes of infectious diseases and their companion fevers, the body's metabolic rate is raised. The body demands more more food, especially more protein, to maintain and repair itself. Thus our Third World human is trying to feed him-

8. The most common parasitic worm of the intestinal tract is the roundworm, *Ascaris lumbriocoides*. It looks rather like a stout 5- to 9-inch-long noodle. Moderate to heavy roundworm burdens are estimated to cause a loss of 15 percent dietary protein and an equal amount of dietary fat. There have been several pilot studies in which children have been treated with several rounds of a cheap, nontoxic anthelminthic (antiworm) drug. Within six months to a year the treated children had an incremental weight gain that was 8 to 20 percent greater than their untreated cohorts. The average cost of the treatment was twenty-five cents per child per year. It would have cost many times that to obtain this magnitude of weight gain by giving food alone to unwormed children.

self *and* his parasites *and* his infectious diseases caused by a multitude of pathogens. The "reference" human of the expert committees and Harvard Scale norms has only to feed himself.

If you don't get enough food, you don't grow as well as those who do. The hungry-looking are not so lean as they are small. One of the first impressions you get when visiting most Third World countries is how little everyone looks. This gestalt of smallness is confirmed when you ask children their age and those you judge to be five or six years old tell you that they are twelve or even fifteen. Despite this, unless it is a famine-struck region one doesn't get a sense of pervasive ill health. Later closer examination will usually reveal cases of kwashiorkor and marsamus but all in all the population, especially in agricultural villages, looks pretty fit. The smallness of stature is not entirely genetic; it is a result of constant, marginal undernutrition. That is, it is undernutrition by our standards. Some would argue that the state of marginal nutrition is not harmful but beneficial. One of the "marginalists" is Dr. John Durnin of the University of Glasgow Institute of Physiology. He and I were participants in a UNESCO interdisciplinary workshop to prepare a state-of-the-knowledge report on tropical forest ecosystems. John was our "nutrition maven" and usually propounded his "minamilist-marginalist" opinions after a sumptuous lunch. We were meeting at UNESCO headquarters in Paris. He came to write in the final report:[9]

There is now convincing evidence that overeating is potentially dangerous; indeed the ideal diet may supply only the minimal necessary quantities of energy and fat, and possibly even protein. . . . There is little doubt that almost any any population of children if fed large quantities of high energy and high protein from

9. *Tropical Forest Ecosystems* (Paris: UNESCO, 1978), ch. 160.

infancy will grow taller and heavier. At the present state of knowledge, it does not seem at all explicit that bigger is better. There are few inherent disadvantages in being small in the physiological sense. Physical working capacity is little altered in absolute terms and, proportionally, is often higher in healthy populations of comparatively low weight.

Current immunological opinion tends to support the nutritional minimalist-marginalists. So far, the *healthy* people of the Third World have been found to develop all the expected, normal immunological repertoire of responses. They can produce the right amount of protective antibody after vaccination. Their cell-mediated immune arm works normally; the T cells are in helper–suppressor balance, produce the right quantities of lymphokines, and the cytotoxic T cells cope with viral and other intracellular infections. It is those who fall below the fragile borderline of mild malnutrition that run into trouble. Gerald Keusch, a knowledgeable immunologist-nutritionist-gastroenterologist of Tufts New England Medical Center, has proposed from his researches in the tropics that immunological responsiveness is adequate as long as an individual is within 60 to 80 percent of the established norm for age and sex of the actuarial tables such as the Harvard-Iowa Scale. Below the somewhat arbitary 60 percent of standard indicates a state of severe PEM.[10] These are the children of the Calcutta streets, the neglected in otherwise healthy villages, populations of drought-stricken West African sahel and Ethiopia, and the peoples starved by war and cataclysm.

The immunological inadequacy of those marked by PEM is reflected in the association, recognized throughout human history, of famine and pestilence. The severely mal-

10. These standards are based on age-to-weight and height-to-weight ratios of a sample of a healthy population. For adults the skin fold thickness which reflects fat stores is another measurement of nutritional status.

nourished are highly susceptible to, and risk being over-whelmed by, infectious diseases. The final cause of death of the starving is usually a bacterial, viral, or parasitic infection. Common childhood diseases, measles and chicken-pox, kill children and adults with PEM. They die of diarrheas and respiratory infections that are rarely fatal in the well nourished.

During the past decade, immunologists have begun to provide the underlying reasons to the clinical observations. To begin with, they noted that the stunting of PEM is within as well as without. Internally there is wastage of muscle and organs. The thymus is one organ so affected and its normal cellular architecture, the area where T cells are processed to maturity, is replaced by fibrous tissue. The starvling's thymus undergoes a premature senile atrophy. As a consequence T cell numbers are reduced and cell-mediated immune defenses diminished. The soldiers of immunity, the phagocytes, don't rally around the invading pathogen in the starved as well as they do in the well nour-ished. Interestingly, once the "starved" phagocytes *do* get to the "sore point," they ingest the bacteria or other path-ogen in normal fashion. However, the ingested pathogen is not digested and killed with the efficiency customary for phagocytosis. Complement levels are also reduced in the acute PEM cases and, therefore, anitbody is less effective in killing invading pathogens.

If we can't get enough food to the famine stricken to allow them to utilize their own immune defenses, can we at least resort to the protective expedient of vaccinating them against the infections to which they are so disas-trously susceptible? The answer is intriguingly confused. Some vaccines protect those with PEM as well as they do the normally nourished while other vaccines afford little or no protection. Vaccines for smallpox, measles, and polio are fully effective in children with kwashiorkor while vaccines for typhoid, influenza, mumps, diphtheria, and yellow fever are not. There are confliciting reports on the use of tetanus vaccine in PEM: some workers have found it to induce protection while others have reported its failure to induce immunity. The reason for the difference in response to vaccines is not clear since even those suffering from severe PEM usually have a normal amount of immunoglobulins in their blood plasma. The B cells seem to be spared in PEM and are doing their thing. What they are not doing in response to some vaccines and pathogens is turning out *specific* immunoglobulin; the product seems to be "rubbish" globulin that doesn't react against pathogen antigens.

There is, however, a dodge to restore immune function when vaccinating the severely malnourished: give them a high-protein diet just before, and a week or two after, immunization. This modest expedient appears simple enough on paper but is probably mostly impossible in the field as any despairing administrator of a famine-relief program is well aware. The tragedy is that it is so difficult to provide enough food to the destitute to bring them even to the threshold of nutrition set by the minimalists' standards. Yet the immune system is so remarkably forgiving that if given an adequate diet, even those with kwashiorkor and marasmus will have their immune system restored to full operating level.

There is, however, one circumstance in which the immune system fails to rebound following nutritional improvement. Should the infant suffer gross nutritional deprivation during the first six to twelve months, the immunological defects appear to be permanent: there is no

restoration even when feeding to full belly pressure is
maintained later in life. In these children there is a persistent thymic deficiency and diminution of cell-mediated
immunity causing them to be particularly vulnerable to
repeated and chronic viral infections. Also, the immune
inheritance of these children is rapidly squandered by
nutritional deprivation. Chapter 5 described how immunoglobulin G (IgG) is transferred from the mother to her
fetus, a passive transaction that will protect the newborn
against the infections to which the mother is immune. The
mother's IgG will persist for approximately two months in
the healthy infant but in the malnourished the turnover is
greatly accelerated and the gift of temporary protection is
lost within a few short weeks. Much later in their life, those
who have suffered infantile malnutrition are more liable to
lymphoma and gastric adenosarcoma cancers.

Even amongst the poorest of the poor, if the babe is
suckled it is nutritionally (and immunologically) protected.
However, there is a growing trend amongst Third World
mothers to follow their Western sisters to the workplace.
In the West, the working mother will usually replace her
mammary absence with a feeding formula that is balanced
in quality and quantity. The Third World working mother
is more likely to feed her infant a cereal gruel that is low in
protein (particularly the highly essential amino acid, lys-
ine), too low in quantity to meet caloric needs, and likely
as not mixed in water contaminated with bacterial and parasitic pathogens. Changing custom, propelled by economic
necessity, is contriving to malnourish and diminish immunity of infants of the Third World.

In many parts of the tropics, infant malnutrition resulting from changing custom is being compounded by chang-

ing agricultural practice of noble intent, the Green Rev-
olution. Before the introduction of Miracle Rice, the peasant farmers grew a mixture of cereals and legumes. The
legumes provided the protein that the cereals lacked and
so gave balance to the diet in agricultural villages. They
were also sufficiently abundant to come within the pur-
chasing power of the urban poor. Comes the (Green) Rev-
olution and there is a labor-intensive, albeit cash-rewarding,
conversion to mono-crop rice farming. The plots of nutritious legumes are either abandoned or so reduced in size
that there is insufficient supply and the market price rises
beyond the reach of the peasant and urban poor. And the
milk-adandoned infants who in former times would have
been compensated with leguminous protein now are more
likely to be given a mono-diet of cereal gruel. Progress has
compromised their nutritional-immunological well-being.

Finally, we must remind ourselves that in the United
States the Third World may be only a few blocks or a short
bus ride away. We have pockets of poverty that almost rival
the worst that the tropics can offer. In 1984, a group of
physicians and public-health professionals went into the field,
visiting eight states in four regions, to examine hunger in
America. They concluded that "hunger is getting worse not
better," an estimated twenty million go hungry at least two
days a month, and in some places charitable food distribution had risen sevenfold within the preceding four years.
The group found American children so affected by hunger
that they suffered from the "tropical diseases" kwashiorkor
and marasmus. Others, somewhat less afflicted, displayed
stunted growth, lethargy, and vitamin deficiencies. These
children of the American poor, immunologically impover-
ished and susceptible to infection, are no longer protected

by the government-sponsored immunization programs. In the United States the infant mortality rate remains higher than in most other industrial nations. The group (the Physicians' Task Force on Hunger in America) recommended that the United States require its own famine relief program at a cost of 5 to 7 billion dollars a year.

# Chapter 10

# Where There's Smoke, There's Immune Depression

TO THE BEST of my recollection, I stuck a pipe in my mouth shortly after my mother removed the teething ring and I had been happily puffing away ever since, along with the burning of an occasional cigarette and cigar. Tobacco, for whatever addictive reason, gave me much pleasure. But it was a mug's game and shortly before embarking on this chapter, I renounced all forms of smoking forever and a day or until my steely will cracks—whichever comes first. Certainly the bad odor of smoking is well deserved. The accumulated evidence leaves no doubt regarding the causal relationship between cigarettes and the modern plagues of industrialized societies—cancer and heart disease—as well as the miseries of the respiratory tract, and, probably, some forms of allergy.

That poet of the dubious and now discounted manly values of sexism and Empire, Rudyard Kipling, is author of the sentiment "a woman is only a woman, but a good cigar is a smoke." Perhaps, but a smoke is also aldehydes, acroleins, nicotine, noxious nitrous oxide and dioxide, phenols, benzyprimines, allergenic protein, and carcinogenic tars. Smoking causes chronic bronchitis, chronic bronchiolitis, emphysema, lung cancer, and cardiovascular diseases up to and including heart attack. Smoking is a powerful immunodepressant that renders both active and passive smokers more susceptible to infection. Rudyard, old man, if you knew what we know today I'm sure you'd reverse your preferences.

The effect of each of the particulate and gaseous components of cigarette smoke on the immune system has not been fully worked out. However, the blanket effect is that it depresses many, if not all, immune functions. To begin the bill of complaint, let us consider the cigarette and the defenses of natural immunity and natural barriers. Unless broken by wounds or abrasions the intact skin covers us quite effectively against pathogens. It is our orifices that are, in the microbiological sense, wide open. Of the orifices, the digestive and respiratory tracts are the most accessible and vulnerable portals of entry for a large variety of pathogens. The respiratory tract is the main juncture where the smoke meets the mucosa. This tract is lined from the nose through the trachea (windpipe) to the large, branching airway passages in the lungs (bronchi) to the small branches (bronchioles) with epithelial cells whose outer surface is covered with numerous, microscopic, hair-like projections (cilia). The cilia trap the bacteria and other particulate foreign matter such as dust, and pollen and, with a kind of rowing motion, push these intruders back up the respiratory tree to where the trachea and gullet meet. Then the bacteria and suchlike, entrapped in a mucous ball, are (gulp!) passed over to the digestive tract to be digested by the stomach acids. In this way, the cilia police the air we breathe and filter out a great deal of the potentially harmful airborne material. Cigarette smoke, particularly nitrous oxide and dioxide in the gaseous phase, acts to impede, or even

totally paralyze, ciliary action. Bacteria and other pathogens escape this first barrier and may survive to establish
an infection. In the case of smokers, the smoke is drawn
into the lungs so that the lower portion of the respiratory
tract (bronchi, bronchioles, and alveoli, the air sacs) becomes
the focus for many infections. In contrast, those who coha-
bit with smokers, in the residential / spatial sense, get their
cigarette smoke, willy-nilly, through the nose. As much as
30 to 40 percent of a burning cigarette's particulate matter
may be deposited in a captive, passive smoker's nasophar-
yngeal passage; for these people the upper respiratory tract
is the site at most risk. For this reason, the children of
smokers are much more prone to upper respiratory infections than the children of nonsmokers.

In the normal course of events on the immune scrimmage line, the macrophages, particularly those located in
the respiratory tract, would act as the second line of natural
defense. The macrophages would recognize every foreign
particle and ingest and digest it. Later, if infection occurs
and antibody is formed, the macrophages would devour the
antibody-coated pathogens with even greater avidity. Several studies have shown that whereas the macrophages in
other parts of a smoker's body look and act normally, those
in the lung are bloated, brown, and filled with matter that
appears to be tobacco gunk. Those lung macrophages give
a very defective performance. They will ingest the bacteria, but their killer instinct seems to have been largely
smoked out: the pathogens remain alive and virulent.

The third type of cell responsible for natural, nonspecific immunity is the natural killer lymphocyte (the NK cell
described in Chapter 8). This specialized lymphocyte,
without any preliminary priming, recognizes viruses and
cancer cells and secretes a toxic substance(s) to kill them.

The NK cells of the chronic smoker appear to be confused; they recognize the viruses and aberrant tumor cells less perceptively and kill less effectively than the NK cells of nonsmokers. Thus, smoking constitutes double jeopardy. The carcinogenic tobacco tars can transform normal body cells to cancer and precancer types and, when these cells *do* arise, the NK cells are less capable to wiping them out. And should the confirmed smoker be so unfortunate as to be stricken with cancer, continued smoking adds a further element of risk. The logic might well be, "What the hell, nothing worse possible can happen, so I might as well allow myself the pleasure and comfort of tobacco." Those who have adopted this crafty logic should think again. It is now evident that continued cigarette smoking by cancer patients compounds the problem. In these people, the cancer is more liable to spread (metastasize) from the primary growth, probably due to the impaired surveillance by the NK cells, than in nonsmoking cancer patients. A cancer that has metastsized is much more difficult to treat surgically, radiologically, and chemotherapeutically.

Specific (antigen-induced) responses are also affected by the dirty weed. Cigarette smokers, especially high-usage, chronic types, have less immunoglobulin G (IgG) in their serum and respond to certain antigen / pathogens with less IgG antibody than nonsmokers. Even amongst heavy users there will be some individuals who appear to be healthy. In the immunological sense the "healthy" heavy smoker is not healthy, despite an apparent ability to produce a normal amount of antibody after—for example—immunization with a flu vaccine. Such a person *still* gets more flu and more secondary respiratory infections than a similarly immunized nonsmoker. Experiments on "smoking" mice have given several clues to the reason for the "healthy but susceptible" problem of human cigarette smokers. If we were to inoculate a mouse with a flu virus and several days later expose it to pneumonia-causing bacteria of such small numbers as to be noninfective, then that mouse would remain alive and well. However, if we were to put the mouse into a smoking apparatus which would have the mouse, poor devil, in effect smoke twenty to thirty cigarettes per day over a period of several weeks and then repeat the same infective procedure, that mouse would die of an over-whelming bacterial pneumonia. Examination of the smoking mouse's immune system would reveal a suboptimal antibody response to both the virus and bacteria, poorly reactive T and B lymphocytes and of course, macrophages derelict in their microbicidal duties. Other smoking-mouse experiments have proved that switching from high-tar to low-tar cigarettes is only partially beneficial. Mice put on high-tar cigarettes in a smoking machine had depressed antibody and cell-mediated immune responses; mice on low-tar cigarettes had normal antibody responses, but the cell-mediated immune arm became subnormally reactive.

For both mouse and man it appears that it takes a lot of smoke over a fairly long period to depress T and B lympho-cyte activity; that is the cell-mediated and humoral immune arms. Two to six weeks for the mouse and two to ten years for the human, at about at least a pack a day. The good news is that the effect doesn't have to be permanent. The immune system, given a chance, is remarkably resilient. Give up smoking and in about six weeks your immune system will be as healthy as a nonsmoker's of your age.

When we are young, disease is an abstraction for most of us. Something we read about, hear about or, if we are biomedical scientists, intellectualize about. Perhaps that is why so many young researchers produce too much that is wonderfully exciting as science but unconnected, unrelated to the pragmatic problems of health and disease. And in the end their findings go nowhere, usually to be replaced by a still brighter isolated scientific nugget of yet another wunderkind. Ah, sour grapes! The effluxion of time brings a harsher reality. Loved ones, friends, sicken and die, and we become more sensitive to the biological clock's chimes of entropy. And so too, a science writer–scientist must write with another character at sixty than he would at twenty-six. Thus, when I come now to write about one of the most common of the dreadful diseases associated with smoking, emphysema, I read my notes but my mind wanders and scans for recollections of those individuals who have played a role in my life; people whom I may not have thought of for years. The personal memory becomes as much a part of reality as the understanding of the underlying immunopathological mechanisms responsible for disease. I remember now a wonderful man, the chief technician of the Protozoology Department of the London School of Hygiene and Tropical Medicine, who taught me so much about my craft. He died many years ago of emphysema.

In the system of Great Britain's post–World War II biomedical graduate education, the Professor occupied a place of Olympian remoteness and the basic "how-to" instruction was mostly given by the departmental chief technologist. During my time at the school, the chief technician was a remarkable man professionally and personally—a combination of regimental sergeant major, teacher, and indulgent mother. He expected both technical perfection and mental flexibility from his predoctoral charges, and on one occasion he had me accompany him to London's East End where we collected a very dead chimpanzee from an animal dealer. Being a frugal man, it was his opinion that taxis were for professors; the tube was more fitting a means of transportation for technicians, students, and dead apes. He wrapped the wretched beast in newspaper (*News of the World,* as I recall), and we carried it to the London Underground. As we boarded the train, with a kind of grand, eccentric nonchalance he put the corpse across our laps. In this way we returned, all the while my mentor describing in clarion tones—smoking one cigarette after another—how it was to be dissected and the parasites extracted. He was a compulsive smoker and when I conjure a memory of him it is of this slight man, peering through smeared, old-fashioned metal-rimmed glasses, the inseparable cigarette in his hand or mouth, and coughing as he smoked. Later, his former students were saddened to learn that he had died of emphysema, although it seemed inevitable that the several daily packets of "coffin nails" would eventually take their toll. Emphysema was a terrible price paid by so kind a man.

Emphysema is primarily a disease of cigarette smokers. It is an obstructive airway disease whose victims suffer from shortness of breath that, in time, becomes a breathlessness on the slightest exertion. The ability of the lungs to function as an oxygenating apparatus fails and the body tissues become increasingly affected by the inadequate amount of oxygen carried to them by the blood. The lungs become vulnerable to infection, and pneumonia is frequently the final cause of death of emphysema patients.

The relationship between cigarette smoking and the underlying immunopathological mechanism responsible for emphysema has only been recently worked out. The scenario according to the new research goes something like this: In addition to particulate matter, cigarette smoke contains glycoproteins, which are antigenic (more about these antigens later). These tobacco antigens are deposited in the deepest recesses of the lungs. The immune system gets the message that foreign proteins and alien particles have come to the lungs, and from the bone marrow's repository a host of monocytes and phagocytic neutrophil leucocytes are sent to the scene to deal with the problem. In time, big smokers come to have big numbers of monocytes and neutrophils in the lungs' air sacs (alveoli). So far so good: these phagocytic cells are acting defensively in scavenging the tobacco-foreign particulate antigen. Unfortunately, a yet unidentified substance in cigarette smoke affects these cells in another way and shifts them into an extra-functional gear. These tobacco-activated macrophages and neutrophils now not only scavenge but also begin to *secrete*. One of their secretions is an enzyme known as *elastase*. Elastase acts like a kind of meat tenderizer that selectively breaks down elastin. Elastin is the tissue material which imparts the necessary elasticity to the air-sac wall to allow it to respond to the inspiration and expiration of air. Elastin is fragmented by the enzyme digestion and these fragments call forth still more macrophages to clear the garbage in the lung. The living body is a remarkable government of checks and balances and under *normal* conditions there is an antienzyme (antiprotease) in the serum which inhibits, or at least limits, elastase activity. However, the second wave of macrophages that come to deal with fragments of lung tissue secrete another kind of substance which inhibits the antiprotease. Now, the inhibitor is inhibited and the elastase can continue to do its digestive dirty work. It takes only six puffs of a cigarette to stimulate the activated macrophages to begin secreting the antiprotease. What begins as a minor breakdown of lung tissue, which can be limited by the body's ability for self-repair, becomes a cascade that digests away the chronic smoker's alveolar walls. The purulent digest collects in, and obstructs, the small tubular airway passages (bronchioles). If the destructive process goes on long enough and too many lung walls come crumbling down then there is, clinically, emphysema. The emphysema-wounded lung is a fertile oasis for bacterial invasion. There are phagocytes aplenty in the lung to cope with the invaders—but remember, the smoker's partially paralyzed phagocytes no longer find the bacteria so ravishingly delectable. Secondary infection is the recurring lot of the emphysemic.

Smoking and allergy has a curious "damned if you do, damned if you don't" relationship. Like all living things, the tobacco plant contains a variety of proteins unique to it; proteins chemically constructed so as to make tobacco tobacco and not a lotus blossom or an armadillo. To a human, tobacco proteins are foreign proteins. They are antigenic. Intimacy with them (and what could be more intimate than drawing them into the deep confines of your body?) produces an immune response. Most chronic smokers do in fact have demonstrable specific antibodies in their blood that react with tobacco antigens. Several of these antigens are glycoproteins, a complex sugar chemically bound to the protein molecule. And glycoprotein antigens tend to be allergenic, eliciting IgE antibody, the immunoglobulin class responsible for immediate allergic hypersensitivity. Once you become allergic to tobacco there is the additional risk of becoming allergic to tomatoes, eggplant, green peppers, and potatoes—all botanic relatives of tobacco, sharing both taxonomic and antigenic characteristics. The antigens of tobacco also show some cross-reactions with the antigens of cocoa, coffee, and ragweed pollen.

As a group, the IgE level in the serum of smokers is significantly higher than in nonsmokers. It is higher still in smokers who are exposed to other environmental allergens. For example, grain handlers (grain dust is highly allergenic) who smoke have much higher serum IgE concentrations than grain handlers who don't smoke. Several convincing studies indicate that cigarette smoking can lead directly or indirectly to allergic conditions, particularly in individuals who are genetically predisposed to react to an antigen in an allergic-immune fashion. It has also been hypothesized that the combinations of tobacco antigens and their specific antibodies (immune complexes) are deposited on the inner wall of the blood vessels of the heart and cause a kind of allergic tissue damage that in time contributes to heart disease. That is the "damned if you do" face of cigarette smoking—Allergic Division.

The "damned if you don't" aspect is an intriguing paradox. If cigarette smoke contains allergens, and if the IgE level is abnormally elevated in smokers, then why is cigarette smoking beneficial in some individuals with one of allergy's most severe forms—asthma? What should we make of the following case histories? *Case:* A thirty-eight-year-old man with asthma since childhood is currently smoking twenty cigarettes a day. He has stopped smoking three times but each time his asthma became so much worse that he had to start smoking again. *Case:* A forty-nine-year-old woman had asthma in infancy which completely disappeared in her teens. She smoked approximately ten cigarettes a day until 1965 when she stopped. A month and a half later she suffered her first adult asthma attack and for long periods thereafter required cortisone treatment to control the severity of the attacks. In 1977, she started smoking again and, within a few months, she was greatly improved and has not needed steroids since.

Case histories of worsening asthma after giving up cigarettes have continued to accumulate. A group of pulmonary specialists became sufficiently impressed by the number and consistency of these anecdotal case histories to undertake a broader, controlled inquiry of their own. These researchers collected a group of fifty-nine asthma patients who had given up smoking and asked them whether they thought that their condition had, as a consequence, improved, worsened, or remained the same. Eighteen patients, 30 percent of the group, reported experiencing a definite deterioration in their condition since they stopped smoking. It was a subjective assessment, but it was an assessment quantitatively confirmed by their increased dependence on medication. Three of these eighteen individuals stated that they had no signs of asthma *until* they stopped smoking. The other forty-one patients experienced no change, for better or for worse. The problem remains as to why all of the group didn't experience a worsening of their condition. Why did renunciation of the cigarette have a deleterious effect on only one-third of the group? Asthma is not a single immunopathological entity but rather a complex of abnormalities. It is possible that the immunodepressant action of cigarette smoke dampens only a limited array of the underlying pathological mechanisms responsible for asthma. Whatever the reason, it would be important to identify the smoking asthmatic who should be cautious in giving up their habit. Or, better still for those people would be the discovery of an agent that would give the same dampening effect as cigarette smoke without the smoke's noxious-toxic attributes.

Another condition in which renouncing, or abstaining from, nicotine has been associated with increased risk and intensification of the disease process is ulcerative colitis. The origins of the notion that smoking has a prophylactic or suppressive effect on ulcerative colitis are in the anecdotal experiences of a number of individuals. Unfortunately, like many other anecdotal accounts in the annals of medicine that bear no statistical clout, the tales of colitis patients were, for many years, ignored. One of my own family members had such an "anecdotal experience." This dear, unfortunate lady was a victim of ulcerative colitis. She was also a heavy smoker—one to two packs a day. Once her condition was diagnosed and brought under control by drugs and diet, she began to feel pretty good again. In fact, she felt so good that she decided to go the whole health route—give up smoking, become a marathon winner, compete at Wimbledon, etc. Within a month of smoking her last cigarette she was in the hospital bleeding from her gut and under threat of surgery. What had gone wrong to cause her fall from the grace of remission? In going over her history with her gastroenterologist, she said that the only different factor in her recent life was that she no longer smoked. And *he* said, "That's funny, I have several patients with ulcerative colitis who have told me the same story."

Another woman had a similar experience but she was the wife of a physician, and he gave her account in a letter to the *British Medical Journal* in 1982. She had been a nonsmoker, but three years after the onset of colitis she began to smoke quite heavily. Within weeks after lighting her first cigarette all her symptoms cleared up. She was, after years of ill health, perfectly well. There was no longer the need for a diet of pureed food and steroid enemas. All was well for another two years, until she heeded the medical wisdom of the day and gave up smoking. Within two weeks all her symptoms reappeared. Her gut ulcerated and bled. The realization came to her that to smoke was to be healthy, but in her mind the cigarette was still offensive. Her husband the doctor substituted the smoke with nicotine-containing chewing gum. The gum worked as well as the cigarette providing she chewed at least five pieces a day, to give a total nicotine intake of 16 to 20 milligrams. Anything less and her bowel relapsed to its former angry ulcerative state.

A few months later another physician wrote to the *British Medical Journal* describing a similar case history, except that his patient had never had signs of colitis until she *stopped* smoking. His patient was a woman who had smoked at least a half a pack of cigarettes a day for the past fifteen years. At the age of thirty-three she quit cold turkey. A few weeks later she noticed blood in her feces, and she began to have frequent explosive, diarrheic episodes—sometimes twenty a day. She was diagnosed as having ulcerative colitis. Demoralized she began smoking again and all the symptoms of the disease disappeared. Eighteen months later she felt healthy enough to give up smoking again. She suffered a relapse several weeks later, began smoking, and became well again.

In 1984 the anecdotes were given a statistical legitimacy (although not everyone believed in the interpretation of the statistics) when a group of British physicians led by Dr. F. A. R. Logan published the findings of their study of 124 patients with ulcerative colitis. As we have noted much of epidemiology is made of premises, premises. Logan et al. assumed that in a "normal" British population (that is, normal in that they had no signs of ulcerative colitis or other bowel disease) age- and sex-matched with their patient group, they would expect to find so many smokers smoking so many fags per day. When they examined the smoking habits of the colitis group, they found there were many more *nonsmokers* than would be expected in a normal, characteristic population. Their statistical conclusion was that cigarette smoking protects against ulcerative colitis and that there is a six times greater risk of developing ulcerative colitis if you are a nonsmoker. Another doctor, K. Amery, looked at the same data and agreed that it was statistically accurate, but that further analysis revealed that *ex-smokers* were even more vulnerable than those who had never smoked.

Peculiarly, for the pathological cousin of ulcerative colitis, Crohn's disease, there is no smoking prophylaxis or relief. As a group, those with Crohn's disease were found to smoke as much, if not more than, the John Q. Public norms.

The immunologic logic for this phenomenon remains elusive. The cause, or causes, of ulcerative colitis are also presently unknown but whatever it is that is destroying the bowel, or causing the bowel to destroy itself, seems to be doing so by an immune-inflammatory process gone amok. The opening passages of this chapter described the many ways that smoking depresses the immune system, particularly the cell-mediated arm involved in the inflammatory process. In all probability, smoking depresses the activity of the destructive immune cells, such as the cytotoxic T lymphocytes, in patients and / or potential patients with ulcerative colitis. (Why it doesn't do so in Crohn's disease, which also seems to be an abnormal inflammatory process, is not even hypothetically accountable.)

So under a few abnormal circumstances, notably asthma and ulcerative colitis, the cigarette may have a beneficial effect in the trade-off with the health risks it imposes. In all other circumstances, smoking is a hazard to your health. It depresses your immune system. It is a mug's game. I can pen these last words with my resolution intact, constant in my renunciation of that evil weed. (If only I wasn't so besieged by sensations of famish. I think I'll see what treasures might be in the fridge.)

# Chapter 11

# AIDS Comes to Our Countrymen: The Problems of Immunodeficiency

AIDS announced itself in America through a rare and exotic parasite, *Pneumocystis carinii*. When the tide of German barbarism finally receded in the last months of World War II it left behind a residue of starving, brutalized peoples. Amongst infants in the nurseries and foundling homes, an epidemic of pneumonia began to occur. This pneumonia was unusual in that the signs of its onset was so insidiously amorphous. The infants first became restless and then went off their feed. Later there was a slight cough, usually accompanied by a sticky mucous expectorate. This gave way to signs of decreasing lung function: their breathing became rapid; they turned blue from lack of oxygen; and ever so slowly, they died. At autopsy the walls of the lung's air sacs, the alveoli, were seen to be grossly thickened and within the alveoli there was a red-staining, honeycomb-like material.

In 1951, the causative organism of this disease, which had become known as interstitial pneumonia, was identified as *Pneumocystis carinii*. *Pneumocystis* is still a taxonomic enigma. It shows some characteristics of yeasts and other characteristics of protozoa. It is capable of infecting a wide range of mammals, although its exact mode of transmission is unknown. It is conjectured that it goes from host to host by airborne suspensions of infective material. The organism may not be so rare as it is silent. Possibly one-third of all humans are infected. Infection does not necessarily mean disease. In the vast majority, *Pneumocystis* remains within us, possibly through much of our life, doing no harm. Nevertheless it is a "sleeping pathogen." Should the infected individual become immunodepressed, deliberately by therapeutic drugs, by malnutrition, or by immunodeficiency disease, this sleeping "yeast-protozoan" will reawaken to pathogenic life, and kill. The malnourished infants it kills slowly. The immunodepressed, particularly older children who are already burdened with the sorrows of leukemia, experience a different clinical course, characterized by sudden onset, spiking fever, and cough. If left untreated, these victims may die within a week of onset.

A number of infections, mostly tropical diseases, are so rare in the United States that their chemotherapies are not subjected to the rigorous and expensive testing procedures required by the Food and Drug Administration. Even so, each year some American citizens—tourists, businessmen, government workers, itinerant scientists—do acquire a nasty exotic. To deal with these cases the Centers for Disease Control (CDC) in Atlanta has established a pharmacological bank of restricted drugs not generally available to the public. Physicians can call this drug bank and have the needed therapy sent to them. In doing so, the doctor has to state the purpose for the drug's use. The data thus accumulated allow government epidemiologists to keep track of the unusual maladies of domestic and foreign origin.

The drug needed to treat *Pneumocystis* interstitial pneumonia, pentamidine, is one such restricted drug available only from the CDC. In this way the CDC epidemiologists knew that *Pneumocystis* pneumonia in the United States is, essentially, a disease of infants under the age of one, and that the average attack rate for this age group is 8.5 per million. That is, *Pneumocystis was* an infant's disease until early in 1979 when the CDC epidemiologists monitoring pentamidine distributions noted that within the past year, shipments of pentamidine had been made to Los Angeles to treat five cases of *Pneumocystis* pneumonia. Epidemiologists must be sensitive to the unusual events and signs that announce outbreaks and epidemics. The epidemiologists at the CDC became alert when they learned from the drug-request forms that this cluster of cases was not of children. All were adults. All were men. They became even more concerned when they learned that all the *Pneumocystis* patients were adult, male, *and* homosexual.

The alarm really went off a short time later when requests for pentamidine to treat male homosexuals with *Pneumocystis* pneumonia began trickling in from New York City and San Francisco. During 1981 and early 1982, each day brought two to five requests to the CDC for pentamidine. Another frightening dimension arose in 1981 when male homosexuals in Los Angeles began to die not only of *Pneumocystis* but also of a rare form of cancer, Kaposi's sarcoma.[1] Also about that time, some male homosexuals died

1. Up to the time of AIDS in America, Kaposi's sarcoma occurred, with very rare exception, only in tropical Africa. East Central African children are at particularly high risk to developing this malignancy. Kaposi's sarcoma begins with lesions of the skin and progresses to invade the lymph nodes, the mucous membranes, gastrointestinal tract, and other organs. In most African patients its progress is slow and if caught in time can be successfully treated by radiotherapy. In AIDS patients, the cancer is much more aggressive and spreads rapidly. However, even in some of these cases it will respond to a combination of radiotherapy and chemotherapy.

of normally minor pathogenic parasitic infections that had become riotously virulent in these patients—*Toxoplasma, Cryptosporidium* (the cause of "scours" in calves and life-threatening diarrhea in AIDS patients), and a bacterium causing tuberculosis in birds, *Mycobacterium avium-intra-cellulare.* By 1983, one thousand gay men, most under the age of forty, were dying each year of one or another of these exotic diseases. The mortality was fearful: 50 to 60 percent of the stricken died within one year. Something was killing the gay males of America.

Such slaughter was completely new to medical experience. If the arts of virology and immunology had been less advanced the shroud of mystery could not have been raised. Early in the search for cause and effect it was realized that underlying this variety of mortal infections and diseases, notably *Pneumocystis* and Kaposi's sarcoma, was a single predisposing factor—immunodeficiency. These killers were known to be opportunistic infections lethal only to those whose immune system had been damaged to impotence.

Some unfortunate people are born with a defective immune system (the primary immunodeficient states). The gays were not born immunodeficient. Their condition, acquired later in life, was thus dubbed *acquired immuno-deficiency syndrome.* To the frightened and helpless it became known by its cruel acronym, *AIDS.* Very gradually a pattern of symptoms came to be recognized as harbingers of AIDS: loss of weight; an underlying feeling of illness; swollen lymph glands; low-grade fever; an episodic diarrhea; an infection, such as a sore throat, that doesn't go away. Feeling under the weather and having a slight fever are no big things to most people, but these same symptoms began to strike terror in the male homosexual community.

Armed with an ability to recognize the early symptoms

of AIDS (the pre-AIDS syndrome) immunologists were able to study the nature of the underlying immune defect before the opportunistic infection took over. This was important because there is a sort of chicken-and-egg problem in the study of AIDS. The immune system becomes depressed and facilitates infection by a microbial pathogen. That pathogen, in turn, further depresses the immune system opening the way to infection by yet other pathogens.

Examination of AIDS and pre-AIDS cases revealed a striking immunological abnormality: a marked decline in the number of helper T cells. The relative absence of the helper lymphocytes left the balance to a preponderance of suppressor T cells. Something seemed to be selectively destroying the helper T lymphocytes, the unit of the immune system so crucial to most defense mechanisms.

The best guess of 1981 was that the killer of helper T cells was a transmissible, infectious agent, probably a virus. This conjecture was supported by the ominous events of 1982. In that year the CDC Exotic Drug facility began to get requests for pentamidine to treat patients with *Pneumocystis* pneumonia who were not male homosexuals. They were hemophiliacs and drug addicts of both sexes. These victims had AIDS and they were *heterosexuals*. The hemophiliacs seemed to be at particularly high risk and this was associated with their life need for blood transfusions. Hemophiliacs are bleeders because they lack a normal blood constitutent, factor VIII, which is essential for blood clotting at wound sites. Factor VIII, prepared from a pooled blood source, is given to hemophiliacs as a prophylactic measure to staunch blood flow in the event of injury. Every case of a hemophiliac who came down with AIDS could be traced to a homosexual donor, a donor that would himself soon have AIDS. Thus, the hemophiliacs contracted AIDS from something transmitted to them by a blood product originating from another individual who was, or was to become, symptomatic. That blood product was bacteriologically sterile, and it was unlikely that it was contaminated with a protozoan parasite. This left the smart money on the viral etiology, and the race was on to find that virus.

The causative virus had to be found in order to devise serological diagnostic tests. It would also be the first step toward a protective vaccine. There were two immediate possible causative candidates—the virus of hepatitis B and the cytomegalovirus (CMV). It was known that many promiscuous gays and drug addicts were infected with these two viruses. However, the epidemiological argument didn't fit the biological fact in that neither of these viruses produced immunological abnormalities characteristic of AIDS. Were there, then, any known viruses of man or beast that preferentially attacked the T lymphocyte?

About ten years ago, in the pre-AIDS age of innocence, my wife and I had a splendid Burmese cat who answered to the name of Supercat. Supercat died of feline leukemia. Feline leukemia is an AIDS-like disease of cats caused by a retrovirus[2] that invades lymphocytes. The feline-leukemia

2. Common knowledge: Viruses are very small, smaller than bacteria, and they cause a variety of diseases in humans, plants, and animals. Viruses are super simple: an inner core of DNA or RNA (the genome), an outer coat of protein (the capsid), and, sometimes, a membranelike lipoprotein envelope. Viruses have no metabolic machinery and are absolutely obliged to live within host cells as biochemical pirates. Viruses reproduce like nothing else on earth. They enter the host cell, losing their outer coat and envelope. The naked strand of viral DNA or RNA genome is the ultimate parasite, it takes over the host cell's metabolism and directs it to produce replicas of the viral genome and capsid. The host cell manufactures other viruses and when this is done, exhausted and damaged, it dies releasing the new viruses to infect other cells. The AIDS virus is classified as a retrovirus, a group of RNA viruses. They replicate by means of an enzyme, reverse transcriptase, which makes a

retrovirus was a class of viruses of warm-blooded animals that fit the bill.

In 1981, when AIDS alarms began to ring, another retrovirus was isolated. This time it was not from a cat but from a human patient with an unusual form of leukemia, a T cell lymphoma. This is a leukemia, a cancer caused by virus-transformed, ever-proliferating T lymphocytes. This virus was given the name *human T cell leukemia (lymphoma) virus I,* which in the taxonomic shorthand of science was reduced to *HTLV-I.* HTLV-I was grown in a T cell tissue culture line and enough virus was harvested to devise serological tests. Application of these tests revealed that about 20 percent of the AIDS patients had antibody specific for HTLV-I. Suspicious? Yes. Convincing? No. The Great Retrovirus Hunt continued.

A year later, in 1982, another retrovirus, different in antigenic character from HTLV-I, was isolated from a human patient suffering from a form of cancer known as hairy-cell leukemia. This virus, named HTLV-II, proved to be another false candidate as the etiological agent of AIDS.

At last, in 1984, four years after AIDS first came into notice, two research groups, one at the Pasteur Institute in Paris led by Dr. F. Barré-Sinoussi, the other at the National Cancer Institute in Bethesda, Maryland, led by Dr. Robert Gallo, simultaneously reported in *Science* that they had discovered the AIDS virus.[3] Each group had taken T lympho-

DNA copy of the viral RNA genome. The DNA copy is integrated into the host's genetic code, which then transcribes for the assembly of new viral RNA and capsid. This is virology in a nutshell. It is also a gross oversimplification, and the interested reader should consult one of the new good microbiology textbooks.

3. In 1983, Dr. Luc Montagnier of the Pasteur Institute described a virus from patients with the pre-AIDS lymphadenopathy syndrome. He named the virus lymphadenopathy-associated virus (LAV) and incrimi-

cytes from AIDS patients and mixed them with an "immortalized" line of T lymphocytes that was being maintained in continuous "test-tube" culture. A virus grew in these cultures and when analyzed showed all the characteristics of a retrovirus and that it was another member of the human T cell leukemia virus family, HTLV-III. For the virologists, these T cell cultures of prolifically replicating HTLV-III became antigen farms. With these antigens it became possible to devise serological tests to determine who was, or had been, infected with the virus. And, in a circular sort of way, provided confirming proof that HTLV-III was the one and only, the true virus of AIDS.

Almost a century ago, the master German bacteriologist Robert Koch laid down the laws for the etiological proof of infectious diseases—Koch's postulates. During Koch's Golden Age of Bacteriology new species of bacteria were being described as the causative agents of disease at almost a weekly rate. Some were true pathogens. Other bacteria were nonpathogenic and happened to be on the scene as part of the natural flora ("flora" because bacteria belong to the plant kingdom). The normal intestine, for example, is chock-a-block full of bacteria. They do no harm and may even do some good in helping to break down food into a digestible, assimilible form. Say you ate a piece of "off" chicken salad at the fireman's Marching and Chowder Society picnic and came down with diarrhea caused by a *Salmonella* bacterium. The bacteriologist would find, in your stool specimen, the *Salmonella* along with a myriad of other bacteria. In Koch's day most of that myriad were still mostly

nated it as the cause of AIDS. There was some doubt about this and his finding was confirmed a year later when it became evident that LAV and HTLV-III were the same virus.

uncharacterized and it was hard to tell the good guys from the bad guys. So how can the researcher say that this particular bacteria or that particular virus is the cause of this particular disease (and get the paper accepted for publication)? Koch demanded two kinds of proof from the claimant of etiological discovery: (1) the organism must be present in all cases of the disease (later, as serological techniques improved, the presence of specific antibody was accepted as a form of proof); and (2) (this is the difficult part) a pure isolate, uncontaminated with any other microorganism, must be inoculated into another, uninfected, human or experimental animal and produce the same disease.

Does HTLV-III satisfy Koch's postulates as the cause of AIDS? Mostly, but not absolutely. The final proof, that of returning the isolated virus to a "clean" human to determine whether typical AIDS would result, obviously cannot be carried out. Nor has the virus yet produced AIDS in experimental animals such as monkeys and chimpanzees. Eventually, Koch's postulate will be satisfied by some careless laboratory worker who will accidentally inject himself or herself with infectious material. Actually, this has already happened. One health worker did get an inadvertent injection of a small amount of blood from an AIDS patient. The health worker developed antibody to HTLV-III, came down with a slight fever, muscle ache, and malaise but, so far, has not developed AIDS or pre-AIDS. This doesn't prove anything, since, as we shall see, it can take as long as five years from the time the virus is acquired to the onset of symptoms. Meanwhile, all the accumulated evidence would have HTLV-III as the causative agent of AIDS.

AIDS and pre-AIDS patients almost invariably have specific antibody to HTLV-III (the few that don't have anti-

body are thought to be so impaired immunologically that
they can't mount an antibody-producing response). HTLV-
III's biological characteristics also support the assumption
that it is the AIDS virus. In "culture-tube" experiments the
only kind of cell HTLV-III will invade, multiply in, and
eventually kill is the helper T lymphocyte.[4] It is the lack of
these helper T cells that is the basis of the immunodeficiency of AIDS.

Thus, it is 99.9 percent certain that HTLV-III is the
cause of AIDS. But is everyone who becomes infected with
HTLV-III invariably destined to develop AIDS? What does
the presence of specific antibody signify? In other infections antibody may be present early in the infection before
symptoms develop, or it may be present after symptoms
develop, or it may be present after the infection is cured.
In some cases antibody can persist for many years, sometimes throughout life. This latter condition reflects a pre-
carious balance in which antibody and other immune
mechanisms haven't got what it takes to effect a sterilizing
cure but are potent enough to confine the pathogen to a
nonvirulent state. Many viruses, such as the herpes virus,
can persist in this live-and-let-live state. In real life, these
questions distil down to: (1) If you have antibody to HTLV-
III, is it a death sentence? and (2) If you have antibody to
HTLV-III, are you, and will you always be, a source of

4. It was first believed that the AIDS virus would only invade helper T
cells and that those cells were the sole reservoir of the virus in the infected
human. It has now been shown that many different types of macrophages can also play host to the virus. It is also now known that 17 to 60
percent of those with AIDS will develop neurological symptoms, which
range from encephalitis to progressive dementia. In a recent paper published in *Science* (September 5, 1986) Dr. Scott Koenig and his colleagues presents evidence from postmortem brains that the neurological
disease in AIDS is caused directly by the HTLV-III virus in the macrophages of the brain.

infection to others? Legitimate questions—to which there are still only inadequate answers.

It is known that:

1. Amongst the healthy male homosexual population a certain percentage are positive for HTLV-III antibody. The percentage differs from country to country, and within gay communities according to sexual habits. In New York City, for example, the serological positivity rate of gays who had been with fewer than ten different partners during the year was 4 percent. In contrast, the group that enjoyed more than fifty different partners per annum (and per anus, since most of the serologically positive are the receptive partners) had a serological positivity rate of 70 percent.

2. Serological testing of several groups of heterosexual hemophiliacs revealed 35 to 75 percent to be positive for HTLV-III antibody.

3. It is estimated that 20 percent of addicted intravenous drug users, male and female, have antibody to the AIDS virus.

4. About 5 percent of healthy, heterosexual Haitian males and females are antibody positive.

5. One study has reported that approximately 20 percent of the adult males in Uganda (all healthy, all heterosexual) were antibody positive.

6. Female prostitutes, especially drug-using female prostitutes, appear to be another risk group. The percentage of serological positivity amongst this occupational group hasn't been thoroughly investigated in the Western world. Rumor in the "microbiological trade" has it that the U.S. Army has carried out a survey for HTLV-III antibody in prosititutes in Bangkok and Manila, two cities where the trade is a cottage industry well patronized by American servicemen. It is said that about 5 percent of the ladies were

found to be antibody positive. My advice to young, male, postdoctoral fellows going to Manila has always been, "Don't even touch the door knobs!" All the newest reports indicate that in several other parts of the world, infection with the AIDS virus is becoming an occupational hazard to the second-oldest profession. A 1986 survey of Haitian prostitutes revealed 49 percent to be infected. They were asymptomatic, but infected nevertheless—and a source of infection to their clients. Similarly high infection rates have been reported in the *femmes libres* in Zaire, and Rwanda in Central Africa.

Suppose you go to the doctor to get a blood test (serology) to find out if you have been infected with HTLV-III and (God forbid!) it comes back positive. Now we come to the Big Question. If there is serological positivity, which is another way of saying that there is, or has been, an infection with the virus, does it mean that AIDS must inevitably follow? It is cold comfort to say that the disease is so new that there is no accurate prognostication. At the time I write this, in the late summer months of 1986, expert opinion holds that AIDS is not the inescapable companion of HTLV-III infection. A few homosexual men have started out, when first examined, with antibody to HTLV-III and became serologically negative six to sixteen months later. These men never developed any clinical symptoms. They presumably became naturally self-cured, in a manner analogous to the immune system's clearing the body of a cold virus.

In Haiti, in Uganda and Zambia, amongst the gays of the Western world, amongst the prostitutes of Southeast Asia, there are, apparently, healthy people walking around with HTLV-III antibody. The present guesstimate is that about 20 percent of the "healthy" serological positives will ultimately develop AIDS. The risk of being a loser in this statistical roulette is highest for promiscuous gays who play the receptive role. This is a "hold-your-breath" statistic and we shall probably have to wait another ten years before the "healthy" antibody positives can be assured that they will have an 80 percent chance of not developing AIDS during their lifetime. The present quandary is that the range of incubation times—that is, the interval between first contracting the virus and the first appearance of symptoms—is not really known. For example, for the flu virus, the incubation period is one to three days, whereas at the other end of the temporal spectrum there is Kuru (the "laughing death" of the Fore people of New Guinea), caused by a "slow virus" with an incubation of ten to twenty years. It seems that HTLV-III can be a fast or a slow virus. Individuals who have received virus-contaminated blood have developed AIDS within months after the infecting transfusion. But the incubation period can be much longer and there is one well-documented case of a tranfusion recipient who came down with AIDS five and one-half years later. Other cases of AIDS may have been incubating as long as eight years. It just hasn't been long enough since the discovery of HTLV-III to determine the outer limit of the incubation period.

Another approach to the problem is to determine whether or not the antibody-positive are also virus-positive. After all, having the antibody has no clinical significance, and is no danger to the public's health if the virus is no longer present. This is a rather new approach and is limited at present because the techniques for isolation, cultivation, and identification of HTLV-III can be carried out only by specialized laboratories. The glimmer so far is that if there is persistent antibody over the years, then the virus also persists, even though the "carrier" may remain in good health.

For that matter, where is the virus in the infected individual, and how is it transmitted from person to person? Again, present information is inadequate. As I noted earlier, it is known that HTLV-III selectively invades and multiplies in helper T lymphocytes and, possibly, also multiplies in the macrophages that it invades. It can, evidently, also be found free in the blood, as evidenced by its presence in derived blood products such as factor VIII. It must also be a rather tough virus to survive the processing and storage of these blood products. Further dissemination of the virus in the body occurs when the infected individual develops the clinical disease of AIDS or pre-AIDS. In these people the virus can be found in almost all the body fluids—tears, saliva, and semen. It is probably also present in the vaginal secretions of infected females. It may also be in the milk of an infected nursing mother.

Despite the virus's wide distribution, the experts maintain that the infection is not easily acquired by those who are not members of a high-risk group. HTLV-III certainly doesn't seem to traffic from person to person like a flu virus: there is no danger in being in the same room with an AIDS patient. This is proved by the fact that there have been no signs of HTLV-III infection in any medical staff attending AIDS patients. The experts maintain that the AIDS virus is transmitted by the intimate avenues of blood transfusion; shared syringes (not only by drug addicts—one case of AIDS occurred in a steroid-using bodybuilder who shared his anabolic-drug syringe with other bodybuilders): abrasive (mostly homosexual) sex; or across the placenta from an infected mother to her embryo. There have now been about a thousand cases of AIDS or pre-AIDS in children. Many of these are orphans—children of drug-addicted mothers who had no symptoms of AIDS at conception, but who developed AIDS after giving birth and died.

This is reassuring to all healthy heterosexuals. Experts discount the possibility that HTLV-III will escape into the general population to become an Andromeda strain. However, the experts haven't satisfactorily explained how those heterosexual Haitian and African men became infected—and since they became infected, why American men are not at risk also. The Haitians, it is suggested, may become infected in voodoo rituals involving scarification and blood. (Or maybe they aren't as inflexibly heterosexual as they claim to be.)

For the Africans, there is hardly any sort of explanation. Maybe they have strange practices we don't know about. Doubtful, very doubtful. Maybe HTLV-III was originally an infection of monkeys and first came to man in Africa. But even if it is a monkey virus there still is no logical explanation of how it came to be transmitted to man if, as it is claimed, intimate contact is needed for transmission. I've known a lot of Africans in my time but none have ever expressed an interest in ravishing an ape. All this makes me a little uneasy. I would agree that HTLV-III doesn't spread from person to person with the ease of a flu virus, but I do believe the potential for HTLV-III to invade the "normal" heterosexuals of the Western world does exist. The notion that heterosexuality will always protect the vast majority from infection with HTLV-III is not necessarily true. Already, several normal, heterosexual wives of hemophiliacs with AIDS have themselves become infected and died of AIDS. The shift in the pattern of infection in Haiti is ominous in that it may portend what could happen in America and Europe. In 1983, over 70 percent of the HTLV-

III positives in Haiti were those in the customary at-risk groups of men—gays, bisexuals, and drug users. In Haiti and elsewhere, promiscuity is associated with the infection but there is that 2 to 5 percent of infections in those whose heterosexual practices are modestly conservative and for whom there is no ready explanation regarding exposure.

There have now been about twenty-eight thousand people diagnosed as having AIDS in the United States (from cases in forty-six states). If the number of cases reported each year are illustrated as a graph, the line from 1980 to 1986 soars steadily upward at an almost 45-degree angle. If that line is extended as a projection of things to come, and if we assume that there will be neither a cure nor significant interruption of transmission, then in 1991 *alone* there will occur 145,000 cases of AIDS in the United States. Also in that year, there will have been, cumulatively, a predicted 270,000 cases resulting in 179,000 deaths that will have cost its victims and the taxpayers somewhere between 8 and 16 billion dollars.

From the beginning, when AIDS was first recognized as a clinical entity, it was abundantly evident that the gay male was most at risk to infection with the virus and the disease. Seventy-five percent of all those with AIDS have been male homosexuals. What were male homosexuals doing that made them so vulnerable? When the researchers came to this perplexing problem, they found that very little was actually known about contemporary homosexual behavior. Gays were like an exotic tribe, with their own customs and habits. What was cousin Bruce *really* doing with that nice young man he lived with? We knew. We didn't know. We didn't want to know. That was before AIDS. Since AIDS, male homosexuals have come under a scrutiny not unlike that which an anthropologist would direct to a "lost tribe" of the Amazonian rain forest. What struck the scientist-observers of the gay scene was that it included a subgroup of highly promiscuous individuals, and that it was these promiscuous gays who were most often being struck down with AIDS. "Promiscuous" is almost an euphemism for the sexual frenzy of that gay group. The sheer number of their partners stuns the monogamous mind: one hundred different partners each month is normal; ten different partners each day is not unusual. I make no moral judgment of this sexual activity except to marvel at it. It does, however, have theoretical bearing on why promiscuous gays are so liable to get AIDS. That they so frequently become infected with HTLV-III is understandable: so many different partners make for a much greater exposure to infection than exists for gays who have monogamous or semimonogamous relationships. No amount of permissiveness about other people's sexual preferences can transform the rectum into a biologically designed sexual tract. It just doesn't have the elasticity and strength of the vagina. No eight-pound baby could enter the world through the anus. Normal heterosexual intercourse does not damage the vagina, but anal intercourse causes small ulcerative abrasions of the rectum. Semen may contain HTLV-III, which can enter the partner's blood system through these abrasions and establish a new infection. I'll elaborate on this in a different context shortly.

It has already been noted that infection with HTLV-III does not inevitably lead to AIDS. Those most likely to have their infection progress to AIDS are the promiscuous gays who are already immunodepressed at the time they acquire the virus infection. Promiscuous gays, even if not infected with HTLV-III, have been shown to have a chronic, low-grade immunodepression. A promiscuous HTLV-III-infected

gay is much more likely to get AIDS than an nonpromis-
cuous HTLV-III-infected gay. This has led to the opinion
that other predisposing, immunodepressing factors con-
tribute to the expression of pathogenicity of the AIDS virus.
The "background" predisposing immunodepression of the
promiscuous gay has been attributed to several different
causes.

Theory A has it that the promiscuous gay's immune system is chronically depressed because they're so often infected
with chronic, sex-related infections such as oral and rectal
gonorrhea and syphilis, the intestinal protozoan parasites
*Entamoeba histolytica* (amoebic dysentery) and *Giardia
lamblia* (giardiasis), and the hepatitis B virus. Chronic
infections with these and other pathogens tend, over a period
of time, to cause a general diminution of immune responsiveness. Then too, genital infections—particularly gonorrhea—attract lymphocytes to the inflamed site. It has been
suggested that the localized concentration of T lymphocytes facilitates infection with HTLV-III; there's a greater
opportunity for virus and T cell host to meet.

Theory B, proposed by Douglas Archer and Walter
Glinsmann, microbiologists at the Food and Drug Administration, is somewhat like Theory A with a nutritional
codicil. Theory B also takes as its starting premise the great
frequency of microbial infection in promiscuous gays.
Approximately 70 percent of all homosexual men engage in
mouth-to-anus foreplay. For the promiscuous gay the variety and frequency of this tongue-in-anus contact infects them
with a greater diversity of microbial pathogens than any-
body else in the world. As a group, the promiscuous gays
have more kinds of pathogenic, or potentially pathogenic,
bacteria in their intestine than a Bangladeshi peasant. Archer
and Glinsmann argue that these constant, polymicrobial

infections will eventually cause permanent damage to the intestinal wall, a wall that has a delicate lining of epithelial cells. It is this epithelial lining that selectively allows nutriments to cross from the intestinal lumen and thence to the body's tissues. The chronic diarrhea that commonly accompanies what has become known as the *gay bowel syndrome* further aggravates the loss of nutriments. This is because there is too rapid a passage of the digested food through the intestine to permit efficient absorption. In time, therefore, the malabsorption, the diarrhea, and the permanently damaged gut tissues result in a state of low-grade chronic malnutrition even when the diet may be nutritionally adequate. Besides, if you're having ten to fifteen "affairs" a day, who's got time to eat properly? Chronic malnutrition, even of a marginal nature, causes a kind of immunodeficiency not unlike that of AIDS itself: a decrease in helper T lymphocyte numbers and a general diminution of functional efficiency of the other specialized cells of the immune system.

Theory B thus proposes that microbial infection causes intestinal damage, which leads to malnutrition / undernutrition, which produces an immunosuppression, which is the "fallow ground" predisposing state that allows HTLV-III to "grab hold" and cause the even-greater immunodeficiency that is AIDS. Archer and Glinsmann are of the opinion that maintaining a high state of nutrition in those at highest risk, even in HTLV-III-infected homosexuals, may be one way of preventing the descent into AIDS. They also note that since there is often permanent, irreparable damage to the gut wall, proper diet by itself may not be a completely effective way to good nutrition and that nutritional supplements may have to be injected or given intravenously.

Theory C is a mite strange, but logical nevertheless. This theory would have it that a large load of sperm in the rectum will induce the immunodepression predisposing to AIDS. Some years ago, it was shown that seminal fluid suppresses immune function. The "depressing" constitutents of sperm are two polyamines,[5] spermine and spermidine. It is hypothesized that these polyamines depress immune function directly—or, step-wise, depress the immune system—to allow activation of two "sleeping" viruses that infect a large proportion of all peoples of the world (of all sexual persuasions): the cytomegalovirus (CMV) and the Epstein-Barr virus (EBV).[6] These viruses, when activated, inflict the aggravated assault on the immune system to open the pathogenic door to HTLV-III.

There is a possible flaw in Theory C's argument. Why should only promiscuous gays be immunosuppressed by sperm? Why not promiscuous females—such as prostitutes—who would, almost daily, also receive a voluminous amount of sperm?[7] The rebuttal by the proponents of the

5. An amine is an amino acid whose COOH group has been enzymatically replaced with an $NH_2$ group. A polyamine is composed of several amines bonded together to form a larger molecule.

6. Forty percent to 90 percent of heterosexuals and about 95 percent of homosexuals have latent (nonclinical) infections with CMV. CMV produces a febrile illness, usually mild in nature, when reactivated in immunodepressed individuals. It can be transmitted from an infected mother to her fetus to produce, among other disorders, severe neurological damage to her child.

EBV is the cause of infectious mononucleosis. It is also incriminated as the causative agent, when accompanied by chronic malaria, of Burkitt's lymphoma. Malaria is thought to be the predisposing factor which allows the EBV to invade B lymphocytes and transform them into unregulated, cancerous growth. Fifty percent to 60 percent of all heterosexuals and about 90 percent of all homosexuals have latent infections of EBV.

7. It first seemed that Haitian females were an exception. They have an unusually high rate of infection with HTLV-III and, in some cases, become

sperm theory of AIDS-predisposing immunodepression is that, histologically, you can't make a silk purse out of a sow's ear. The tissue structure of the vagina and the rectum are very different. The vagina is lined with a thick, stratified layer of epithelial cells that resists abrasive injury and confines sperm to the vaginal tract. In contrast, the rectum is lined with a single, delicate layer of epithelial cells. Sperm polyamines are capable of passing through this layer to make contact with the cells of the immune system present in the deeper tissues of the bowel wall. The bowel lining is also liable to ulcerating damage by anal intercourse, which would allow still further exposure of the blood and lymphatics to sperm.

Which of the three theories is correct? Probably all three theories are correct in part. It is also highly probable that there are still other predisposing factors of AIDS yet to be discovered.

A vengeful (white, male, heterosexual) God most certainly did not create HTLV-III in 1979 to smite the sinning gays. In an earlier book, *New Guinea Tapeworms and Jewish Grandmothers* (Norton, 1981), I contemplated the origins of certain infectious diseases—Lassa fever, legionnaire's disease, babesiosis—that seemed to be completely new to human experience. It seemed to me that these strange infections were spewed up from some seething witch's cauldron. However, while the conspiracy theory of infectious disease is attractive, it's not very logical; I concluded that these diseases came lately to man because of altered behavioral, ecological, and / or environmental conditions that brought the pathogen, from animals or other humans, into

stricken with AIDS. Careful inquiry into Haitian sexual behavior revealed that Haitian women and men frequently resorted to anal intercourse as a birth-control measure.

more widespread and intimate contact with the population at large. For most of these "new" infections a pattern of epidemiological events could be traced.

Now amongst us comes HTLV-III and AIDS. The origins of AIDS are so unclear that one is almost repersuaded to demonic epidemiology. It does not seem to be an infection that has actually been present in the Western world for many years unrecognized by medical science. For one thing, the AIDS syndrome is so clinically dramatic that all but the dimmest physician would have been aware of its presence. For another, there is a sizeable collection of serum taken from hemophiliacs more than ten years ago and since preserved by deep freeze. None of those sera has been found positive for HTLV-III antibody: there is no sign of infection. Now, as you know, 35 to 75 percent of hemophiliacs are, or have been, infected with HTLV-III.

AIDS theoreticians would have it that the ancestral home of HTLV-III is East Central Africa, and that the virus has been present in humans there for hundreds, if not thousands, of years. They say that AIDS cases have occurred in tropical Africa in the past and have gone undiagnosed because of the thin, overworked medical services there and because AIDS as a clinical entity was obscured by the great number and variety of diseases common in African peoples.

Serum samples taken in Africa during past epidemiological surveys and stored by deep freeze don't go back very far in time. The earliest samples from Central and East Africa are from the early 1950s. Recent serological reexamination of these sera showed several to be positive for the HTLV-III virus. In Europe, where the medical services are good and AIDS can be identified, many, if not most, of the AIDS patients have been heterosexual African immigrants. For example, in 1983 thirty-five of the thirty-eight AIDS patients in Belgium were African immigrants. The few seroepide-miological studies carried out in Africa lend support to the African AIDS Homeland notion. One population living in a remote area of Zaire had a 12 percent positivity rate for antibody to the AIDS virus, with the highest rate in young children. None of these people, adults or children, showed any signs or symptoms of AIDS. All were within what is considered to be the health norm for an African villager. This first led to the belief that in Africa HTLV-III may really be an infection of children in whom it runs a relatively mild clinical course terminating in self-cure, like measles. And like measles the virus can be deadly when it infects adults who are "immunological virgins," as measles has been when introduced to the Eskimos or pertussis (whooping cough) to the tribesmen of the western New Guinea highlands. Unexplained is how the children acquire the infection if it is, as it is believed to be, transmitted sexually or by blood transfusion. Perhaps it is in the milk of infected mothers. Perhaps it crosses the placenta and the infants are born with HTLV-III.

Africa has been the Dark Continent as far as informa-tion about AIDS is concerned. Until 1985 very little data had come from East and Central African countries—areas where AIDS is known to be present and, possibly, pre-valent. Quite frankly, the African researchers had been stonewalling the issue. They have cancelled presentations or walked out of scientific meetings when the question of AIDS in Africans was brought up. It has been a politically sensitive subject, but by 1985 the situation had so deterio-rated that disclosure became necessary. AIDS, in its var-ious guises, has come to East and Central Africa. All indi-cations are that in this part of Africa the HTLV-III virus is now expressing itself with the same virulence seen in the

Western world. The difference between America and Africa is that in Africa most of the cases are promiscuous heterosexual males and females. In Uganda there is a syndrome of AIDS characterized by rapid weight loss. The condition is sufficiently common that the Ugandans have given it the sobriquet "slim disease."

Also unexplained is "Why now?" Why didn't HTLV-III migrate from Africa to the West many years ago, especially during the colonial era when there were many whites in black Africa? Believe me, the Colonial Service recruited a few homosexuals along with the majority of heterosexuals. During my time in the British Colonial Service in Nigeria, I knew several district officers who preferred the company of the village lads to that of the nubile village lasses. They were tolerated as eccentrics (particularly so if they were graduates of Oxford or Cambridge) who were to be kept in the bush and not posted to administrative centers. One macho, big-game hunting, polo-playing assistant district officer in a town I visited during the course of sleeping-sickness research was famous throughout the province. Three sheets to the wind on champagne he would make a midnight ride, bareback and bare assed, two-up with his African male love of the moment. He performed this ritual at full gallop through the streets of the town, blowing his fox-hunting horn all the while. He never got AIDS (although I did hear later that the Queen gave him the Order of the British Empire). Nor did the gays of the French, German, Belgian, Spanish, or Portuguese colonial services. If HTLV-III and AIDS truly sprang from Africa there is still a missing link to the story, and I wonder if it will ever be found.

At the moment the prospect of cleansing the world of AIDS is wintry bleak. Asia and the Pacific basin have, so far, been spared but it is doubtful that these regions can long remain isolated from the infection.[8] In the Americas, in Europe, and in Africa the number of cases increases, sometimes doubling, with each passing year. As I have already noted, the cases are mostly gays but there are frightening signs that the infection is escaping into the heterosexual population. True, it does not seem to be transmitted by "judicious" sexual behavior or proximity. Sex may have begun with a protozoan but many million years later it is "omnipresent . . . woven into the texture of our man or woman's body."[9] Sexually transmitted pathogens are wonderfully successful in sustaining their continuity. Herpes lives! And God help us if HTLV-III mutates to become the herpes of the eighties or nineties. HTLV-III kills.

We can't look foward to the chemotherapeutic "magic bullet" pill for succor. Chemotherapy research has yet to gift mankind with any practical, effective drug to combat any viral disease—let alone AIDS. The antibiotic your physician gives you when you get a "virus that's going around" is to prevent secondary bacterial infection or to give you the impression that something is being done for the thirty-dollar office visit. Any virus. Any antibiotic.

The best hope is that an immunizing vaccine can be developed. The inability to infect and produce AIDS in experimental animals seriously impedes vaccine research. It is not sufficient to extract an antigen from a killed virus and "shoot up" those at risk: that antigen may provoke anti-

8. HTLV-III has not, so far, been transmitted within Japan. Many Japanese hemophiliacs, perhaps 50 percent, have antibody to HTLV-III and several have been stricken with AIDS, but this has been from American blood products. The Japanese seem to be reluctant blood donors and they import 300,000 liters of blood and blood products from the United States each year. They sell us Toyotas and we send them blood. What could be fairer?

9. Havelock Ellis in the *New Spirit* (New York: Boni and Liveright, Modern Library edition, n.d.)

body formation and still not be immunogenically protective. Determining which antigen preparation, if any, is protective and safe for use requires arduous research best screened in experimental animals. Genetic engineering that would create a microbial centaur—a bacteria expressing an HTLV-III antigen—is a future possibility. I would conjecture that it will be five to ten years before the first shots of a licensed vaccine are given. And if HTLV-III turns out to be a "flighty" virus given to mutating to new antigenic types, analogous to the flu virus, then a vaccine may never become a practical reality.

Other clinical-research workers have faced the facts of life—and death—that there are no therapeutic measures against the virus and that the best immediate hope is to treat the immune system itself to return it to working order. A serious immunological defect is the inability of AIDS patients to produce the lymphokine, interleukin 2. Interleuken 2 is the lymphokine secreted by activated helper T lymphocytes which stimulates additional helper T lymphocytes to proliferate and differentiate into a "working" force. Interleukin 2 also stimulates the lymphocytes to produce gamma interferon. It is gamma interferon that prompts and enhances the cytotoxic T lymphocytes (the killer T cells) to attack virus-infected cells and zotz the virus within them. Both interleukin 2 and gamma interferon can now be harvested in pure form by immunological and genetic engineering techniques. Both substances are currently being given, on an experimental basis, to AIDS patients. So far, the trials have shown them to be of some, but not terrific, value. Perhaps they will be more efficacious when optimal doses and regimens have been worked out. Nor is it known whether their activity is transient, palliative only so long as they are being injected, or will be therapeutic in helping the helper T lymphocytes return to permanent health.

Organ transplant? The immune system can be considered as an organ, even though its cellular components are disseminated throughout the body. Operatively, an immune system transplant would be much simpler than a heart transplant: a simple injection of lymphocytes or bone marrow from a healthy donor. But foreign organ tissue is foreign organ tissue be it lymphocyte or liver, and it will be rejected. And since there still would be an ongoing virus infection to invade the new T lymphocytes—even if they did colonize in the recipient patient—this form of treatment doesn't appear promising. In one case the tissues were perfectly matched and it still did not help the AIDS-stricken patient. In this unusual case one of a pair of identical twins got AIDS while his brother remained uninfected with HTLV-III. Identical twins derive from a single, split fertilized egg and are, therefore, identical in all antigenic attributes. Their parts, given an available operative technique, can be interchanged. Lymphocytes and bone marrow were transferred from the healthy to the sick twin, whose condition began to improve. Then, as the virus attacked the new cells, the stricken twin deteriorated and he died.

Money for AIDS research is not lacking. Congress appropriated $233 million for 1986 to cover all AIDS-related activities. About half of this is to go for research. The Public Health Service has asked for $351 million for 1987 and $471 million for 1988. Research money helps but it doesn't guarantee discovering a cure—the economics of cancer research has taught us that. Crash research programs do not mean that the best minds will be bought and brought to the problem being sponsored. There's nothing quite like a sudden treasure of big research bucks to bring the hacks out of the woodwork. Undoubtedly all the new money will buy a mass of information. A small amount of it may even be therapeutically applicable, but the bulk will be the minutiae beloved by scientists. All this is a way of saying that within the next few years we are going to learn a great deal about HTLV-III and AIDS but don't expect too much in the way of a cure.

Neither vaccine, nor drug, nor biological stratagem can now stay the course of AIDS. But if not curable, AIDS is largely preventable. Traditionally, preventive medicine—the least traumatic and the most sensible and effective way of maintaining health—is the least respected and rewarding of the medical specialties. Preventive medicine works by the individual doing most of the work. This too frequently requires relinquishing cherished, ingrained bad habits—be they unwholesome habits of food or of sex. None of us like to give up these goodies and, under ordinary circumstances, few of us are able to do so with constant resolve. However, it may just be that AIDS has so frightened the more promiscuous of the gay community that they will adopt a new life-style. One sign of that change was related to me by an acquaintance who is gay. The romantic homosexual ideal has been, since the days of ancient Greece, the willowy young man. Today the willowy young homosexual is the most likely candidate to get AIDS (and if he's *very* thin he already may have the disease). My friend tells me that the former beau ideal has been replaced by the statistically safer fat and forty-ish type. Most gays do recognize the need for preventive behavior—and if not celibate, they are becoming much more circumspect and more monogamous in their relationships. One healthy sign is that between 1980 and 1984, rectal gonorrhea in San Francisco male homosexuals declined by 73 percent. This is a marker of behavioral change. It is a sign of engagement with fewer partners and conversion to more prudent sexual practices. But not all homosexuals have become converts to prudence. There is a hard core—the bathhouse crowd—whose habits do not appear to have altered. In late 1983, investigators from the University of California–San Francisco AIDS Behavioral Research Project questioned homosexual men in bathhouses, bars, non-frequenters of bars or bathhouses, and those with a committed monogamous relationship. All but the bathhouse group said that during the AIDS eighties they had reduced their visits to, or had completely stopped frequenting, bars and bathhouses. The bathhouse group hadn't, for the most part, changed their life-style although they were well aware of the risks. The investigators concluded that this was a fatalistic, addictive behavioral pattern. There was a discrepancy between understanding and behavior: "Sexual behavior may be comparable to other high-risk behaviors such as tobacco smoking, obesity, non-seat-belt use, and alcohol consumption, where knowledge alone is not sufficient to change behavior."

Effective measures to prevent AIDS in that other highly vulnerable group, the hemophiliacs, have already been implemented. Blood donors are being serologically screened, and rejected if found positive. Stored blood and blood products are also being serologically tested and the HTLV-III contaminated stock destroyed. This should prevent new cases from occurring in hemophiliacs and others who require blood transfusions. The present increase in the number of cases probably represents, to a large degree, old, latent infections becoming clinically patent. With care, judicious

sexual behavior, and great good luck there will be a dramatic decline in the number of new cases after the current
AIDS victims have passed from the scene. Prevention will
have to be vigilant and perservering—it is estimated that
there are at least one million HTLV-III carriers—Typhoid
Marys of AIDS—in the world today who could start the
disease cycle again, and again.

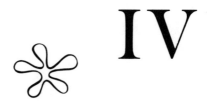

# IV

*The Future of Immunity
and Immunity in Your Future*

# Chapter 12

# Psychoimmunology: Id, Ego, and Lymphocyte

IT IS the year 2000. In the psychiatrist's office a patient is reciting a familiar litany. "My business is in shambles. My wife and I fight constantly. I am at the brink of bankruptcy and divorce. I'm enraged at the world but can't vent my feelings. I feel awful, I have boils, and if there is a cold going around within fifty miles, I'll catch it."

"I am here to shrink your troubles," says the future shrink. "We'll talk; meanwhile here's a prescription for pills to smooth your mood. Also, from the laboratory tests I see that your depression has had a bad effect on your immune system and I am going to give you another prescription for medicine that will be an immune tonic. We know now that there is a kind of dialogue between your psyche and your immune system and, therefore, your treatment will be psychoimmunotherapeutic."

Another year-2000 patient has cancer and is being treated by an oncologist, a nutritionist, and a psychoimmunologist. The psychoimmunologist is a new breed of medical professional. He is monitoring the patient's immunological profile and treating him by behavioral conditioning, using a procedure descended from Dr. Pavlov's dogs salivating at the ring of a bell. The behavioral conditioning has improved the patient's immune response that is fighting the cancer and has also allowed for a reduction in the amount of the toxic anticancer drugs that have to be given.

That the mind is of the body has been realized ever since humans began to contemplate on the nature of their emotions and their illnesses—the "psychosomatic medicine" of moderns. Repeated studies have confirmed that the life expectancy of the bereaved husband or wife is frequently shortened after the death of their spouse. For over twenty years a British scientist, G. W. Brown, has studied the relationship of tribulations he understatedly calls *life events*—bankruptcy, imprisonment, relocation, etc.—to illness. He found that those subjugated by these life events had significantly more illness and a higher mortality rate than age- and sex-matched controls whose life sailed on a more even keel.

If a life event makes for greater susceptibility to disease it means that it is somehow impairing the immune system. During the 1950s and 1960s experimentalists began attempting to mimic human travails in the life of a mouse to determine their effects on the immune response. Instead of bankruptcy and bereavement, the life event inflicted on the mouse was a series of inescapable shocks. The immunological effect depended on the nature of the shock. Mice given big shocks produced less than the normal amount of antibody after being injected with a standardized antigen, whereas low-shocked mice produced more than the normal amount of antibody. Later mouse-shockers, who knew more about the intricacies of the immune system, found that the big, inescapable electric shock caused lowered T lymphocyte and natural killer (NK) cell function. NK cells are concerned with controlling the spread of cancers, and the shocked mice had a significantly shorter survival time after implantation of a mouse mammary cancer than normal control mice, or mice that had been given lower levels of electric shock which they were given the opportunity to avoid.

However, electric shock isn't exactly a customary human life event, even for electricians, and investigators began to explore experimental designs that were more "human" in circumstance. In one such experiment, monkeys that had been together as a socially bonded group since birth were separated. Within weeks of their being isolated, T cell numbers and function declined. When the monkeys were restored to the group their T cells were restored to full number and activity.

Finally humans came under the psychoimmunologist's scrutiny. At Mount Sinai School of Medicine, investigators sought to discern the effect of profound grief brought on by the impending death of a loved wife on the surviving husband's immune system. The T cells of fifteen men whose wives were terminally ill with advanced breast cancer were found to be less than normal in number and impaired in function. The men had an immune profile not unlike the monkeys saddened by their loss. The possibility of other, contributing factors was largely ruled out: the men had maintained a customary diet as reflected by an unchanged weight. They carried on with their usual activities and did not become anemic.

If mood and emotion can so depress the immune system, is the reverse true? Can we laugh and psychologically "catharsitize" our way out of sickness? This is a very new concept and very few investigations have been carried out on psychological intervention as a form of immunotherapy. One pioneering study in this area has been carried out by Dr. Sandra Levy and her colleagues at the University of

Pittsburgh School of Medicine. Her group compared the psychological type and immunological status of cancer patients with little lymph node involvement (favorable prognosis) to that of cancer patients with extensive lymph node involvement (grave prognosis). The latter group was psychologically characterized as being apathetic. They were deemed to be emotionally paralyzed by suppressed rage. Immunologically, their natural killer cell activity was, functionally, also apathetic. In contrast, the psychological and immunological status of the patients with little or no lymph node metastases was "healthier." They were of brighter disposition, able to ventilate their feelings, and their immunological functions—notably NK cell activity—appeared to be normal. In deciding on cause and effect, the obvious question that arises from the Levy study is which came first, the advanced cancer or the apathy? Did the apathy cause the cancer to be more aggressive or did the advanced cancer bring on the apathy? Behavioral intervention studies now in progress are attempting to answer this question. Cancer patients with a personality profile considered to be associated with immune dysfunction and rapid deterioration of their condition are being given supportive psychotherapy to determine if this results in a clinical-immunological improvement.

Nor does a life event have to be as ominous as cancer or imprisonment to be immunodepressive. At Ohio State University, medical students studying for their final examinations were found to have T cells that gave subnormal responses to antigens and mitogens. Come to think of it, teachers know that there are an uncommonly large number of "I am sick, excuse my absence at the examination and please arrange for a makeup" messages at exams time. Obviously, what will be a life event for one person may be only a stimulating experience for another person. It is for the psychoimmunologists of the future to determine the characteristics that make a personality type susceptible to life's immunodepressing experiences and also to define the variety of those experiences.

One of the most fascinating potential clinical applications of psychoimmunology has come from the serendipitous observations of an experimental psychologist, Dr. Robert Ader. Ader was studying how rats could be conditioned for taste aversion. The behavioral conditioning technique was essentially like that of Pavlov, who rang a bell each time he fed a dog: after a time the dogs salivated in gustatory anticipation at the bell's ring even though no food was given. For his conditioned reflex experiments, Ader gave rats water containing saccharine, whose sweetness pleasured them. When the rats were "hooked" on the sweetwater he injected them with cyclophosphamide immediately after each time they drank. Cyclophosphamide rapidly causes nausea in the rat and Ader wanted to find out how many nauseating experiences were necessary before the rats developed a learned aversion to saccharine water. After the aversion had been solidly established, Ader stopped giving the cyclophosphamide, in order to determine how long it would take before the rats returned to drinking saccharine water again.

In human terms, Ader's experiment can be described in the following way. Suppose you had an uncontrollable desire for cherry cheesecake (a not unreasonable uncontrollable desire) and your doctor deemed that for health reasons you must go cold turkey on cheesecake. The habit might be broken by giving you a pill that would make you nauseated after the first bite of cheesecake. Eventually you would be conditioned so that the very sight of cheesecake would make you sick to your stomach. However, without a reinforcing nausea-inducing pill now and then you would probably relapse into your old cheesecake habit. And that is what happened to Ader's rats: they returned to drinking saccharine water avidly again. But something else happened to those rats—they began to die from infections and cancers. This occurred long after they had received the last injection of cyclophosphamide, and there was no apparent reason for the abnormally high mortality.

Ader enlisted the help of an immunologist colleague, Nicholas Cohen, to solve the riddle of the dying rats. Cohen quickly found that the dying, behaviorally conditioned rats had markedly defective cellular (T cell) and humoral (antibody–B cell) immunity. The startling implication of this finding was that not only had behavior (saccharine-water avoidance) become a conditioned response but the immune response had also been reflexily conditioned. A conditioned reflex had been established in which the nervous system was controlling the function of the immune system. The Pavlovian bell rang and the T cell stopped functioning.

For his avoidance-conditioning experiments Ader wanted a drug to bring on a quick nausea, and cyclophosphamide fulfilled that requirement. What Ader the psychologist may not have realized—as did Cohen the immunologist—was that cyclophosphamide is a powerful immunodepressent that appears to work by inhibiting the replication of cells such as transformed lymphocytes and tumor cells. So, along with the nausea, Ader was inducing a transient immunodepression. What was not anticipated was that the immune system is under "mind control" (in ways that are mechanistically not well understood), and that long after the rats forgot their learned aversion to saccharine water the immunological conditioning continued to "remember." Drinking saccharine water had become a stimulus of the conditioned reflex by which the central nervous system dampened the immune responses. It was a stimulus that remained intact after the behavioral conditioning had faded.

Ader and Cohen have envisaged several situations in which modification of the immune response by behavioral conditioning could have clinical application for the treatment of human diseases. One possibility would be for the treatment of autoimmune diseases such as systemic lupus erythematosus (SLE)—conditions in which a deranged immune system is destroying the body of the person to which it belongs. Presently, treatment of SLE and other autoimmune diseases consists of giving powerful immunodepressive drugs such as cyclophosphamide. These drugs are toxic, and the patient is precariously balanced between the drug's toxicity and the disease's pathogenicity. Mice have their own version of SLE. It too can be treated with cyclophosphamide. Recent research has shown that, after behaviorally conditioning SLE-afflicted mice with saccharine and cyclophosphamide (à la Ader), it was possible to therapeutically immunodepress the animals with the saccharine stimulus alone. Actually controlling the disease in the behaviorally conditioned mice still required cyclophosphamide, but 50 percent less drug was needed than for the control (unconditioned) mice with SLE. The extension of this research would be to try to behaviorally modulate human patients whose immune system needs to be dampened: those receiving organ transplants; those suffering from autoimmune disease; and, possibly, those with certain types of lymphoid cancers.

Equally intriguing is the prospect that behavioral conditioning could enhance immune function of normal, healthy humans to provide a strengthened prophylactic defense against disease. During illness, the immune system sends disaster signals to the central nervous system. The brain and other components of the central nervous system respond by helping formulate, in ways still imperfectly understood, the strategy of the immune response—by directing the traffic of the cells of the immune system, for example. That phenomenon (the message received and replied to) is feedback. However, there is another, lesser known, phenomenon—feedforward. In feedforward, the reply is made before the message-stimulus is received. An example of feedforward is the response in people who strenuously exercise regularly. The stress of exercise causes the body to accommodate to the demand by increasing heart rate and blood flow, to increase adrenalin output to get the competitive spirit in train. If the exercise is routine, a feedforward conditioning is established—the very anticipation of the exercise is all that is required to get the juices flowing. The heart rate and the adrenalin level are increased *before* you enter the track, the tennis court, or the aerobic exercise class. With this in mind, psychoimmunology researchers are beginning to ask: If Ader and Cohen could behaviorally depress the immune system with an immunodepressive drug as one element of the conditioning process, why can't the immune system be enhanced by using immunostimulants in a similar way?

The use of immunostimulating drugs may not even be necessary in behaviorally conditioning the immune system. Remember the rats who were given a "tingling" shock from which they could escape? Those rats had a heightened immune response; they produced more antibody than "normal" control rats after a single injection of an antigen. Are there analogous "low-shock tingling" stimuli that we humans could be given to boost the immune response in a similar fashion? Does pleasure foster immunity? If we laugh uproariously at a Marx brothers movie, are our B cells and T cells also delighted in the functional sense? And if so, could they in time be conditioned to respond by our merely seeing a photograph of Groucho? Big issues for big thinkers.

From the foregoing, I submit that there is abundant evidence that the immune system is influenced by the mind. One immunologist, J. Edwin Blalock, goes so far as to argue the case for the immune system being a sensory organ, like the eyes and ears. However, for the scientist the observation of mind over immune matter is not enough. The real challenge, the real fun, and where the research funding is to be found is in how the immune system works. From studies on the relationship of the immune and nervous systems, several biochemical pathways have been discerned, the foremost of which involves the body's response to a life event, to stress.

Beginning in the mid-1930s, physiologists and rat-shocker psychologists, led by Hans Selye, began to look at the "slings and arrows" in terms of stress. Physiologists-endocrinologists elucidated, by what is now considered to be classical research studies, a hormonal cascade in rats acutely stressed by repeated unavoidable electric shocks and in humans stressed by great life events. In this cascade, the hypothalamus[1] responds to the imaged signal of stress by producing and secreting a substance called *corticotropin releasing factor*. The releasing factor, in turn, signals the pituitary gland (an anatomical neighbor of the hypothalamus) to pro-

1. The hypothalamus is a collection of cells located deep within the forebrain. It is a primitive structure with regulatory and hormonal secreting functions. It responds to primitive, basic stimuli: hunger, thirst, libido, rage.

duce a hormone known as *adrenocorticotropic hormone (ACTH)*. ACTH circulates in the bloodstream and targets to the adrenal gland and biochemically "instructs" that gland to manufacture and secrete corticosteroids. Thus, pharmacologically, a stressing experience is akin to corticosteroid therapy.

The immunosuppressive activity of steroids is well known. Few of us reach ripe maturity without having been given steroids for some inflammatory condition, which may range from tennis elbow to ulcerative colitis. Despite long and widespread use, surprisingly little is known regarding the actual mechanism by which the steroids inhibit the immune response. The latest theory, for which there is quite good evidence, is that the corticosteroid doesn't work directly on the lymphocyte but rather redirects the traffic of the T and B cells from the bloodstream back to the bone marrow where they remain inertly unresponsive to the calls for immune action.

Corticosteroid is not the only immunodepressive substance produced by the stressed individual. Stress literally drugs the immune system into submission. You may recall the publicity some years ago of the finding that the brain, in response to stress, produces a substance whose activity and chemical structure is remarkably similar to that of morphine. This neuronal secretion (really a family of substances collectively known as opioid peptides) was given the name *endorphin.*

Clinical and experimental investigations have shown that human morphine addicts and mice experimentally made to be addicted are more susceptible to infectious diseases, have a higher rate of cancer than is normal for their age and sex group, and tend to suffer abnormally accelerated tumor growth. This is much like the pattern of vulnerability of those mice and men immunodepressed by intolerable stress. Although the explanatory research is still in its relative infancy, it has been found that opioid peptides inhibit lymphocyte function. The natural killer cell seems to become particularly "stoned" by the opioids, and this could account for the higher cancer rate and the uncontrolled aggressiveness of the tumors. Similar to the stimuli evoking corticosteroid production, mild, escapable stress does not induce the neuronal cells to secrete opioids: it takes big, continuous stress for the mind- and immune-numbing morphoids to be called forth.

This literary journey began in the bucolic countryside of eighteenth-century England and ends, in a sense, in the office of a twenty-first-century psychiatrist. The ending reflects the growing appreciation that the immune system is of the body. Its workings are as influenced by emotions, nutrition, inheritance, and environment as any other of the body's organ systems. In this integrated way science will continue to instruct us how to make the most of our immune system. The promise is that we will have new vaccines, new immunomodulating drugs, new nutritional strategies, and new means of "self-control" by behavioral conditioning. The promise of the future is that we will live with immunity.

# Chapter 13

# Promises, Promises

SCIENTISTS looking into the crystal ball risk being dazzled by their own reflection, and this can seriously limit their ability to prognosticate. Biomedical science is a restless, opportunistic endeavor: a succession of modish disciplines, each promising to provide the golden highway to health and long life. As the fashion of the discipline fades, some important, practical tangibles remain from the blaze of ideas, the mountain of publication, the largesse of funding. Obviously, the discipline doesn't actually expire; research continues—albeit at a more subdued level—and some devotees remain at work in the field, like memory lymphocytes that can be revitalized by restimulation. The problem is that during the discipline's peak fermentive period it is often difficult, if not impossible, to discern what is "vain foresight" from what will become established benefices.

We are now in the midst of immunology's Imperial Period. It is currently the dominant biomedical "ology." All the other "ologies" including, as we have noted, psychology / psychiatry pay tribute to it. Molecular biology, virology, parasitology, and oncology are only a few of the disciplines whose current major research efforts are directed to immunological aspects.

Each day we learn more about the workings of the immune system. There is so much seductively fascinating new knowledge that it becomes difficult to discriminate what is important in a "where-the-rubber-meets-the-road" way: the findings that eventually will be of practical benefit.

On reflection, I may be overly sensitive to this issue because of a personal feverish experience. Man and boy, during some thirty years of research in tropical climes I never had malaria. I took my pills, slept under a mosquito net, and led a prophylactically charmed life. Then, in 1984, when I was working in Papua New Guinea on an aspect of immunity to malaria (Do fetuses of malarious mothers become immunologically "primed" while in the uterus?), that charmed life came to an end. We (my wife, myself, and a marvelously comical hornbill with Bette Davis eyes named Bubbie) were living in Goroka, a highland town where malaria doesn't much occur (it's too cold at night for the parasite to survive inside the mosquito). It was on one of those cold highland nights, two weeks after I returned from a field trip to the Southern (and malarious) Gulf region, that the ague struck: paroxysms of shivering followed by drenching sweats and brain-wracking headache. These were the symptoms that I had for years described to my students as being the high drama of the malaria attack. I took a course of the prescribed therapeutic drug, chloroquine, and felt quite well within a few days. Two weeks later, in the midst of a breakfast conversation with Bubbie on the merits of a papaya we were sharing, the icy chill from that wretched parasite (a particularly lethal variety as the microscope later revealed) struck again. It was resistant to all the conventional modern drugs, and the only treatment was to return to the four-hundred-year-old nostrum, quinine.

It may be that malaria makes for a confused mental state, but my reaction to the episode, as the fever broke, was one of irritation and indignation.

Twenty years before, when I had last worked on malaria in New Guinea, I would have never become infected. The parasite was fully sensitive to chloroquine, a cheap, relatively nontoxic drug. DDT—a cheap, nontoxic (to humans) insecticide—was sending millions of mosquitoes to the Big Blood Meal in the Sky. Malaria was being brought under control, and there were good prospects for its global eradication. By 1984 the parasites had become resistant to almost every drug but quinine and the anopheline mosquitoes thumbed their palps, so to speak, at the insecticides sprayed at them. There was more malaria in New Guinea in 1984 than 1962. And what is true of New Guinea is now true for almost all of the tropical world.

In the years between 1962 and 1984, scientists were assiduously unlocking the innermost secrets of the malaria parasite—the detailed complexity of the immune response, how to grow the parasite in the test tube, the molecular mechanisms of its chemical physiology—illuminating the minutest feature of its morphology. My file of reprints was bursting at the seams. I had even contributed a few ounces to the total tonnage of publication. And yet, despite that Leviathan of information, with each passing year, we were less able to deal with malaria *pro bono publico*. So, as I sweated, felt god-awful, and my ears rang from the quinine, I thought, "I'd trade the lot of you molecular biologists and T cell immunologists for one good Ehrlich-type who could come up with a new drug and / or insecticide." In that sentiment, I would be joined by the majority of "working" malariologists throughout the tropics.

Now that I am defervesced and again ensconced in my

laboratory, surrounded by all my toys and graduate students, I realize that this attitude is largely one of scientific boobism. And I am chastened. But I am also realistic, and I advocate caution and discrimination in judging what is, and what will be, good medicine for you and me and Everyman. Or put another way, don't be blinded by science. Having said that I will now place my bets in the Immunological Sweepstakes.

## Big Ideas for Old Shots

It would be tempting and certainly better show business to begin the immunological prognostications with high-technology portents—synthetic and recombinant vaccines, monoclonal antibody-targeted carriers, immunomodulators. In reality the greatest immunological benefits will probably come from the tried-and-true, well-established vaccines. These are the vaccines which we in the industrialized West have been immunized by and see to it (or should see to it) that our children are also immunized by.

On the other side of the world, in the shanty cities of compressed humanity and in the dirt-poor countryside of Asia and Africa, there are some 800 million people with a yearly income of less than $150 who live on the thin margin of starvation and disease. For these people improved health services and, many authorities insist, improved educational services (particularly for females) are the two essentials to be met before quantity, the proliferation in population numbers, will be traded for quality, the better life for a population whose growth has been controlled.

Some ninety million children are born each year in what is euphemistically called the Developing World. The vital statistics are faulty and undoubtedly underestimated,[1] but of that number some fifteen million will die during their first year of life, six million of these from infectious diseases. They die from diseases preventable by immunization. In addition to the deaths, one of every two thousand children born in the Third World will become lamed by polio.

It is a terrible, needless human waste. And, I assure you, mothers mourn their dead children in an African village as deeply as mothers do in the Western world. To bring a halt to this killing, the World Health Organization in 1974 proposed an Expanded Program on Immunization, which aimed at immunizing all the world's children, by 1990, against six diseases that now cause five million deaths each year in the tropics: diptheria, pertussis (whooping cough), tetanus, measles, polio, and tuberculosis. The vaccines were

1. In the tropics you really can't believe all that you read on the charts adorning the health ministers' office walls. Many of the statistics on life, death, and disease rates shown on those charts are derived from information furnished by the rural primary health centers. These centers do the best they can but often as not they don't have good intelligence as to who is sick, or who has died or been born in the villages which they service. As an example: Not long ago I was an advisor to several Asian countries on the control of kala-azar (a particularly nasty sandfly-transmitted protozoan disease of the tropics and subtropics). In the capital cities the statistical sections of health ministries give me precise numbers of cases occurring each month and where they are occurring. Where do the numbers come from? They come from the monthly reports sent to them by the district health centers. I go for a ride in the country, to the district health centers. The physicians and health assistants at all the centers tell me that they haven't had stocks of the curative drug for the past several years. The local people are painfully aware of the situation. They also know the distinctive symptoms of kala-azar and when they become ill very few go to the health center because they also know they won't be treated. Those with money go to private practitioners who don't have to report the disease to government authorities. Those without money stay home and die. After a few days in the field it was obvious that the incidence of the disease was being egregiously underreported.

available. They were of proven efficacy and safety (although the BCG immunization against tuberculosis is a bit iffy as to its efficacy,[2] and there is some question as to the safety of the pertussis vaccine). And they were cheap: vaccines for all six diseases would cost a mere seventy cents. Moreover, even if it wasn't possible to immunize everyone, there should still be a beneficial ripple effect if a large enough proportion of the children could be vaccinated. In that case there would be so few infections—and, consequently, transmission from person to person so reduced—that even the unvaccinated would be at little risk.

The Expanded Program on Immunization progresses each year. Even so, a dozen years after inception of the scheme less than a quarter of the Third World's children have been immunized. There have been problems. Let me describe a day in the life of a person we will call Nurul Chakrovarty, a vaccinator of a country we will call Xenostarkia.

Nurul Chakrovarty is twenty-two years old and an educated man. He has had seven years schooling, reads and writes in Xenostarkian, and speaks some English. He can do sums and keep records. Two years ago, the government hired him to be a vaccinator in its Expanded Program on Immunization. They trained him for three months, during

2. BCG is Bacillus of Calmette and Guerin—an inactivated strain of *Mycobacterium bovis*—the cause of bovine tuberculosis. It is claimed that it has sufficient antigenic similarity to the human tuberculosis pathogen, *Mycobacterium tuberculosis,* to afford protection. This has been debated; some studies have shown that it works while other studies have shown it to be useless. In the largest and latest trial, in India in 1979, which involved 260,000 people half of which were given BCG and the other half a placebo vaccination, BCG proved to be completely ineffective. There have been criticisms as to the design of that trial and defenders of BCG say that the variability in response relates to variation in potency between different batches of vaccine. For now, the World Health Organization advises playing safe and giving BCG.

which time he was taught how to transport the vaccine, the crucial necessity being to maintain the cold chain—that is, to keep the vaccines at the proper cool, preserving temperature. He was taught how to give shots, schedule immunizations, and keep proper records. He was also taught a little about the diseases he was to protect the children against with the vaccines. Nurul understood all this very well, except maybe the diseases part. Those lectures were given by the World Health Organization consultant, an affable Yugoslavian who spoke no Xenostarkian and whose strangely accented English confused Nurul.

On this day Nurul had to travel to a health center about ninety miles away from the capital city: not prohibitively far, but there was a large river to cross by ferry and the last twenty miles was more of a track than a road. Fortunately, this was the dry season. During the monsoon the track was impassable even by four-wheel-drive vehicle and Nurul had to slog those last miles, burdened with the cold box containing the vaccines and the inoculation supplies. The plan today was to make an early start: to be on the road by 6 A.M. At six Ali, the driver, was somewhere in the bazaar having an early-morning cup of tea; Musa, the assistant vaccinator, was also somewhere in the bazaar having a wake-up bowl of rice; and Zakir, the bearer, who had to walk five miles from his home, hadn't arrived yet. By half past seven everyone was assembled, the vaccines stored in the cold boxes, and the boxes containing the syringes, needles, records, and other paraphenalia loaded into the Landcruiser. By great good luck (and a small bribe to the dispatcher in the motor pool) Nurul was allotted that day a reasonably new vehicle, one that had been given to the immunization program by a European government less than a year ago. Most of the vehicles were roughly used and poorly maintained. His poor government didn't have the sponduliks (the basic unit of Xenostarkian currency) to buy spare parts, so they were inoperable a good deal of the time. One of the few project vehicles that was in good condition was used by the Director to take him to and from work (but that is as it should be, the Director is an important man). At least Nurul had gasoline for this trip. Last month he couldn't make his appointed rounds because the project ran out of the gasoline money that had been budgeted for that month. He couldn't complain, though—his friend Naryan in the malaria program hadn't been out of the city for eight months because their budgeted fuel allocation had been exhausted early in the year.

Nurul and his team arrived at the river's edge two hours later, and after a half hour the ferry pulled up to the dock. So far all was well. On Nurul's last visit to this village the ferrymen went on strike while on the other side of the river, and the ferry didn't appear for two days. Meanwhile his vaccines had lost their cool. Nurul didn't know if they were any good when he finally got to inject the children.

The river crossing never failed to delight Nurul. In the cool breeze the sailing barges with their flamboyantly colored sails floated by like great, lazy birdwing butterflies. The ferry held a lively community of its own: food vendors, entertainers, even healers. For a few sponduliks Nurul had a healer rub a snake skin (with the snake still in it) over his ankle, which had been giving him trouble. Already his ankle felt better. Would that all medicines were so simple and effective.

By noon they had reached the other side of the river and Ali, one hand never leaving the horn, was taking them over the road at a furious pace. Ali despised his vehicular inferiors, the bicycle rickshaws and oxcarts that crowded the road. Today, the cursed Ali actually hit a rickshaw. It took a half hour in the hot sun, with the vaccines slowly warming, to sort out the altercation. Those rickshaw wallahs have no respect for government men.

A little after half past one they arrived at the health center. Too late. The health clinic doctor had already left for his private practice in town. What else could the poor doctor sahib do? The government paid him a mere two thousand sponduliks (fifty dollars) a month. He had to see paying patients each afternoon so he could live in at least the minimal style befitting a doctor. Even so, about 150 mothers with their children had assembled and were patiently waiting on the health clinic's veranda. Doctor or no doctor they would have to be attended to. Nurul was disappointed that only 150 mothers had come. Children of 500 mothers were scheduled to be inoculated. He scolded the clinic's health auxillary wallah whose job it was to make the rounds of the district's villages informing the mothers that the vaccinator would be at the clinic on this day. The health auxillary explained that the soil was being prepared for planting, and many of the women whose labor was needed in the fields couldn't afford to walk those hours to the clinic, then wait at the clinic until they were attended to, and then walk back to their village. The headman at Mubai village, that ignorant peasant, told his people that the vaccinations would make the children ill. Most of the mothers from that village wouldn't come. Then, last week when he was supposed to visit the northernmost villages of the district his motorbike broke down once again, so those people never got the message.

These people are impossible, Nurul thought—always excuses. But he must get to work. He opened the cold box containing the vaccines. A quick inspection showed that the temperature-sensitive piece of tape hadn't changed color: the vaccines were safe. Although he now knew it by heart, Nurul made a confirmatory check of the immunization schedule printed on the card he carried.

| AGE OF CHILD | IMMUNIZATION(S) |
|---|---|
| 3–5 months | BCG, 1st diptheria-pertussis-tetanus (DPT), 1st polio |
| 6–8 months | 2nd DPT, 2nd polio |
| 9–10 months | 3rd DPT, 3rd polio, measles |

Whenever possible he tried to vaccinate pregnant mothers with tetanus toxoid during the second half of pregnancy.[3] So many babies died of tetanus if the mothers were not immunized.

Each mother carried the medical record of her child, on which the immunizations given, if any, were entered. It never failed to surprise and please Nurul to see how carefully the village mothers protected the cards from the rain, rodents, and roaches.

Musa and Zakir unpacked the supplies of sterilized needles, syringes, and alcohol swabs, and got to work. Some children screamed when they were injected, while others remained stoically silent (probably the ill or malnourished ones, Nurul thought). A few records were mixed up. A few children had had their names changed since the previous round of immunizations and that also confused the record

3. When pregnant mothers are immunized they will form IgG antibody (as will, of course, nonpregnant women). This antibody will then cross the placenta to accumulate in the developing fetus's blood. Thus the newborn infant will have a passively acquired antibody that for the first few months of life will give protection against tetanus. Neonatal tetanus, which has a mortality rate of 80 percent, is common in the Third World due to the unsterile conditions and practices surrounding birth.

keeping. It was the custom amongst the people in this district to change their name if an illness or some other misfortune occurred. It was also customary to deny that the person with the former name ever existed. This fooled the Fates. It also fooled the health personnel (and, sometimes, the tax collector). Otherwise all went well. By five that afternoon all the children had been given their immunizations. A little gossip, a cup of tea, and the immunization team was on the road to make the last ferry of the day. They arrived back in the city a little after ten that night, tired, very tired, and with an endless round of health clinics to be visited on the days to come.

The vaccines Nurul used cost seventy cents for each child. To that seventy cents, administrative costs added another nine dollars.

While the World Health Organization was advocating the immunization program to halt the needless deaths of Third World children, America also remembered its sickly past. In 1921 there were in America some 200,000 cases of diptheria; in 1934, 250,000 cases of whooping cough; in 1941, 900,000 cases of measles; in 1952, 21,000 cases of polio; and in 1968, 150,000 cases of mumps.[4] By 1982 the widespread immunizations given to children had reduced the yearly incidences to 3 cases of diphtheria, 1,500 cases each of measles and whooping cough, 5,000 cases of mumps, and 7 cases of polio (three of which were caused by the vaccine, a rare untoward occurrence). All this and more (tetanus and rubella are also included in the standard immunizing regime)

4. These dates are given because they are the years when the respective diseases were first made legally notifiable; i.e., the doctor was required by law to notify the health authorities of each case that they had diagnosed. Thus, these are the years when the first accurate data on the incidence of the disease became available.

for a total cost of about ten dollars per child for all immunizations. There has never been a greater bargain.

In 1974 the Surgeon General of the United States announced national goals for the continuing immunization of America—goals that were projected to be achieved by 1990. That program is not only working, it is ahead of schedule. It is just possible that by 1990, or shortly thereafter, measles and polio will become extinct in the United States—historical curiosities.

This splendid achievement has come about through good vaccines and enlightened legislation. It is now the law in all fifty states that each child must have had all immunizations in order to enter primary school. Federal largesse has helped. Washington has been steadfastly generous in funding (with our tax dollars, of course) immunization programs for children of the poor. At present, about half the immunizations are given by private doctors to paying patients and the other half given, mostly to poor families, at local and state health clinics. However, our immunization program is in peril. Its is beset by budget cutters who would rather buy pork barrels than vaccines. Ultimately, I think reason will prevail; public concern will insure that our tax dollars will continue to protect our children.

In fact, lawyers may be a greater danger to the immunization program than the budget cutters. Very few products in this world can be guaranteed to be absolutely safe. This is as true for vaccines as it is for your family car. Vaccines are being continuously improved for safety and potency. Even so, for reasons that are still obscure, some untoward and severe effects do occur in a very few individuals. The pertussis vaccine has been particularly liable to give rise to adverse side reactions. Of the 13.5 million pertussis immunizations given in the United States 43 of them have caused death or severe brain damage. This is hardly a satisfactory state of affairs, but it seems a reasonable trade-off for protection against a disease that in some parts of the world has a mortality rate of one in fifty.

Parents of children who have been killed, or physically or mentally crippled by a vaccine, sue. And prompted by their lawyers they sue big. The children and parents get a lot of money and so do the lawyers. If a pharmaceutical company is faced with $50 million in vaccine-related litigation they are in big trouble. More and more of these companies are saying the hell with it—there's not that much money in vaccines anyway. Vaccine production is being curtailed or abandoned by these manufacturers, creating the threat of vaccine shortage—a shortage that will prevent attainment and maintenance of the 1990 health goals.

No matter how excellent the vaccines, there will always be some small risk associated with immunizations. Even so, the overriding consideration for public safety demands that childhood immunizations should be mandatory and that suppliers who have met all the regulatory requirements in the manufacture of a vaccine should not be penalized for the rare "act of God" mishaps. When pertussis immunizations dropped in Japan and England because of the concern over adverse side reactions, epidemics of whooping cough followed within one to two years. It seems to me that our society must rethink the whole issue of crime and punishment as it applies to medical care. The federal government has to some extent assumed the role of guardian of public safety, interpreting the Constitution as a mandate for them to do so. They assumed that role in the 1970s during the swine-flu fiasco by paying the claims of those who had suffered a severe untoward reaction to the vaccine and were suing the manufacturer. This was a step in the right direction, even if it was more of the same. The claims were paid except that this time it was with tax dollars.

And yet, the public will swallow all kinds of snake oil proffered by the eccentrics and quacks and some will sicken and some will die as a consequence. Rarely will the quacks be taken to court by their victims.

We can't have it both ways. Medical progress and medical care has its price tag of misadventure. Based upon the best of available knowledge, regulatory agencies such as the Food and Drug Administration try to keep that price tag as low as possible. It may even be that these agencies have set the price so low, by insisting on so many exhaustively restrictive proofs, that medical progress is being impeded to a disproportionate degree. We must do the best we rationally can and take our lumps along with it, suing the vaccine manufacturer only when there is a criminal deviation from the licensed production procedure. In those cases the punishment should fit the crime.

Legal and logistic problems notwithstanding, the future augurs immunologically well for the world's children. That's great, but us old folks are also at risk to infectious diseases which are preventable by immunizations. Influenza is the first of these infections that come to mind. We all know how terrible one feels when down with the flu and how many working days are lost. People over sixty or sixty-five may lose more than a few days in bed: they can lose their life. In the grand scheme of vaccination goals for the 1990s and the new century we grown-ups haven't been forgotten. Our national policy, for starters, is to have at least 60 percent of those at greatest risk to severe influenza, notably the aged, be given annual immunizations. At present only about 20 percent of the at-risk groups are being immunized despite the vaccines having become more potent, more type-specific, and freer of adverse reactions since the swine-flu days. It might also be noted that at present Medicare does not pay for influenza immunizations for the aged.

Rubella, alias the German measles, is a mild viral disease occurring mostly in children and young adults. The great danger from rubella is that if the infection occurs during pregnancy the virus can cross the placenta to infect the fetus, in which case it will cause severe abnormalities—brain damage, heart disease, deaf-mutism, cataracts. The mother who has had rubella before becoming pregnant is immune and cannot become reinfected to pass the virus to her developing embryo. However, 15 to 20 percent of American girls come to reproductive age (in an earlier, starchier time they would have described as being of "marriageable age") without ever having had rubella. These women are at greatest risk during the years when rubella comes in epidemic proportions. Two such years were 1964 and 1965; in that period 20,000 babies were born with congenital rubella-caused defects, and 6,250 fetal deaths, 2,100 neonatal deaths, and 5,000 therapeutic abortions, occurred.

There is an effective rubella vaccine made from an attenuated virus.[5] A single immunization affords a protective immunity for at least sixteen years and, probably, for life. The vaccine is usually formulated as a combination of mumps, measles, and rubella (the MMR vaccine) and is being given to children as a requirement for primary school entrance. The 1990 goal is to have at least 90 percent of the

5. Immunization with rubella vaccine, or any vaccine made of a live attenuated virus, must be done before pregnancy. Immunization with these vaccines during pregnancy is dangerous. The vaccine-virus is capable of crossing the placenta to infect the fetus and even though attenuated and nonvirulent to the mother it may cause harm to the child she is carrying.

children immunized with MMR by the age of five and 95 percent by the age of twelve. Meanwhile all women contemplating pregnancy would be well advised to be tested to see if they are immune to rubella, and if not, to be vaccinated before they commit themselves to motherhood. If childhood and adult immunizations are carried out as planned and if there is no complacent faltering in the immunization program, by the year 2000 the rubella virus may join the smallpox virus in the deep-freeze vaults that store pathogenic microbial relics.

Hepatitis B (serum hepatitis) is bad news for adults, but a protective vaccine is now available. However, an immunizing dose costs one hundred dollars. Hepatitis B, a viral infection, usually causes only a mildly symptomatic infection in children who make an unremarkable recovery and become asymptomatic carriers of the virus for the rest of their life. In contrast, adults who acquire the infection (usually from a transfusion of blood from a carrier donor or, in the case of drug addicts, from shared syringes) develop a fulminant hepatitis from which the mortality rate is 10 percent higher. Most survivors recover completely, although about 10 percent become carriers. There is convincing evidence that the chronic carrier state in adults can lead to liver cirrhosis and liver cancer.

The hepatitis B virus cannot, as yet, be grown in tissue cultures so there is no "antigen farm" to make a vaccine. However, there is an antigen, a viral particle, in the blood of human carriers, and by processing large amounts of that blood a vaccine can be prepared. It is an expensive process, hence the hundred-dollar immunizing price tag. Because of the cost and the limited amount of vaccine available, it is now being given to those most at risk, such as medical personnel, including medical students, who are in danger from an accidental stick with a contaminated syringe needle, and to those who for medical reasons must have repeated blood transfusions. Few drug addicts are being immunized, although they belong to the group most likely to become infected. A better, cheaper vaccine is needed and high technology is addressing that problem with remarkable success. And it is with those high-tech advances that I will begin the prognostications for the next generation of vaccines: the immunizations that are in our future.

## New Shots from New Ideas

Basically, vaccines haven't changed much since Pasteur's day. Pathogens are killed or attenuated, tested for safety and potency in animals, and that's the vaccine. I predict that the immunizers of the twenty-first century will look back on this era as the Stone Age of Vaccination. The next generation of vaccines will be prepared by entirely novel means and allow immunization against a variety of infections for which we now have no prophylactic measures except judicious behavior or the constant pill (as for gonorrhea and malaria, respectively). The two emerging mainstreams of the new vaccine technology are genetic engineering, the recombinant-gene methods, and man-made synthesis of vaccines.

All living things—plants and pandas, ameobae and anthropoids—are an assemblage of protein molecules. Even a bacterium is composed of hundreds, or thousands, of different kinds of protein. Each of those different proteins would be antigenic; each would elicit a specific immune response. A different antibody, for example, to each protein antigen. In the past, vaccines have been made from whole organisms, the entire antigenic assemblage, that have been modified in some way to render them nonpathogenic. For many microbial vaccines this technique has worked: the vaccines have been protective. For other pathogens, whole-organism vaccines have not done the job.

It may be difficult to grasp because of the confusion of terms, but the fact is that not every immune response is a *protective* immune response. Not every antigen is an immunogen (an antigen that induces protective immunity). Thus, we might inoculate an antigen of a bacterium into a mouse and the mouse would do all the expected immunological things: it would produce a specific antibody to the antigen and mount a specific cell-mediated (T cell) response. And yet, when that mouse would be challenged with an inoculum of the living, virulent bacteria, it would sicken and die. Its immune response would not have been the kind that was protective. However, when another antigen from the same bacterium would be injected into another mouse the response, in that case, would be protective. The mouse would be truly immune in the actual as well as the semantic sense. There are even some antigens that when given with the "good antigen" (the immunogen) would interfere with the development of the desired protective immunity.

The reasons why one particular antigen and the response it elicits from the immune system is protective while another antigen and the response it evokes is not are not well understood. For the moment, for all practical purposes it is enough to know which antigen is protective and to have the technical know-how to extract it in pure form from the molecular mass that is the whole microbe. There is a growing list of "pure" immunogens isolated from viral, bacterial, and parasitic pathogens. Importantly, a number of immunogens are from microbial pathogens for which vaccines had not been successful. Many immunologists now believe that ultimately only pure immunogens will be used as vaccines.

Genetic engineering now makes the concept of the "pure immunogen vaccine" imminently possible. The immunogen is a protein constructed from instructions of the genetic (DNA) code. Biotechnology now has the methods to (1) identify and locate the gene which codes for the wanted immunogen; (2) snip out that bit of the DNA code; and (3) insert that DNA sequence into the bacterium *Escherichia coli*, or the yeast that makes your bread, *Sacchromyces cerevesiae*. So now we have these two harmless microorganisms, growing prolifically in a simple culture medium, who in the genetic sense think they are, for example, a hepatitis B virus antigen and instruct their RNA to assemble the viral immunogen that will be used as a vaccine.

The making of a hepatitis B vaccine has been a pioneer objective of this kind of genetic engineering. A recombinant-gene-produced vaccine which is the same antigen as that found in the blood of carriers is now under trial in chimpanzees (one of the few experimental animals that are susceptible, in human fashion, to hepatitis B). These trials have indicated the recombinant vaccine to be protective, but it had the same limitations common to all recombinant-gene-produced vaccines designed for human use. Along with the desired antigen there is also all that extraneous material from the yeast or bacterium. This extraneous material, which itself is antigenic, can produce an adverse hypersensitivity effect when injected (especially when it is repeatedly injected) into humans. Existing legal restrictions for vaccine licensure require that the vaccine be free from all the potentially harmful extraneous matter, and the purifying techniques do not yet exist.

*Nil desperandum!* say another group of genetic engineer-immunologists. There is even a shrewder solution to the problem. Not only is the extraneous matter a limitation of a recombinant gene vaccine from a bacterium or yeast, but also that vaccine is a dead vaccine—a nonliving antigen. The immunizing effect of a dead vaccine is relatively short-lived, and periodic restimulation by revaccination is necessary to maintain a protective immunity. The answer, propose the genetic engineers, is to insert the desired antigen-coding segment of DNA not into a bacterium or yeast but into a completely benign microorganism which will live in the human body for long periods, preferably for life, and have that microorganism constantly manufacture the protective antigen. All well and good, but what microorganism fulfills the criteria to be the DNA carrier? That microorganism, reply the recombinant mavens, is available, and has been available for more than two hundred years—the vaccina virus that has faithfully and benignly immunized the world against smallpox. When first attempted, the technique for inserting a viral antigen gene into another virus (the vaccina virus) proved to be somewhat trickier than recombinant insertions into bacteria and yeasts. The methodology has finally been worked out and some immunologists foresee unlimited possibilities in creating vaccina-delivering vaccines.[6] Vaccina-hepatitis B, vaccina-influenza, and vaccina-herpes vaccines have been developed and are now in the animal-testing phase. The vaccina-hepatitis B vaccine has protected chimpanzees and has, so far, produced no adverse effects. If and when this vaccine comes into the public domain the cost of immunization against

6. "Vaccina-delivering vaccines" appears to be tautological. To be strictly semantic, vaccine means an immunization with vaccina virus (cowpox virus—Latin *vaccinus*, "of or from cows"). Modern usage is somewhat anti-semantic in that vaccine has come to mean, generically, all the antigens used to induce a protective immunity.

hepatitis B is expected to be reduced from the present one hundred dollars to thirty cents.

Then there is a third group of neo-immunologists who predict a dead future for vaccines derived from living microorganisms. This group of scientists say "Why use these old-fashioned vaccines at all when we can manufacture—from scratch and in unlimited quantity—vaccines that will be purer, more potent, and much cheaper?" For over twenty years the immunochemists have been assembling, Tinker-toy-fashion, chains of amino acids that were specifically antigenic when attached to a carrier protein. These experiments with the synthetic "nonsense" antigens revealed that a chain of ten to twenty amino acids acted as an antigenic determinant and a substitution of as few as one or two amino acids caused major changes in biologic properties. Recently, it was shown that what was true for the synthetics held true for the natural antigens—their determinants (epitopes) were also restricted to a short sequence of amino acids in their protein molecule. New techniques made it possible to identify the location of the critical sequence, snip it out of the chain, and, finally, to analyze it for its amino acid composition and the order the amino acids were strung together. With this knowledge it became a relatively simple matter of taking down the needed amino acids from the shelf and assembling the epitope in the test tube.

Epitope manufacture is at an early stage of development although immunochemists see limitless possibilities for this approach to vaccine production. Already, a synthetic hepatitis B vaccine consisting of thirty-eight amino acids bound to a carrier protein[7] has protected some (but

7. Remember Chapter 5; only a small chain consisting of ten to twenty amino acids is involved in specificity but a big, weighty chain (of which the small chain is a part) is required to switch on the immune response.

not all) of a group of chimpanzees against the disease. Synthetic epitope vaccines of influenza viruses, polio viruses, and the diptheria toxoid have elicited the kinds and concentrations of antibodies in rabbits and other laboratory animals that are associated with immune protection, but those vaccines have not yet been put on trial in humans.

One of the more intriguing experimental synthetic vaccines now on the human horizon is one that has been assembled to immunize against malaria. Immunization of humans against malaria has been a goal of parasitologists since 1912. All sorts of experimental vaccines have been contrived to protect birds, rodents, and monkeys against *their* malaria but so far no vaccine can protect humans against theirs. While the drugs and insecticides were doing what they were supposed to do there wasn't any great need for a vaccine, and research on the subject languished. However, now that we have largely lost those chemical strings to our bow the search for a malaria vaccine has been revitalized by a large infusion of interest and money.

A major obstacle to developing a malaria vaccine relates to the complexity of the parasite's life cycle. A bacterium is a bacterium all its life and remains morphologically and antigenically constant. In contrast, a malaria parasite, as it progresses in its cycle from the mosquito to the warm-blooded host, is a gamete, a zygote, an ookinete, a sporozoite, a trophozoite, a schizont, a merozoite, and a gametocyte.[8]

8. Gametes, male and female, are the equivalent of the egg and sperm of higher life forms. The zygote is formed by the fusion of the male and female gametes. The zygote enlarges to form the ookinete which in turn divides to form the sporozoites, the infective stage. All these stages are in the mosquito phase of the malaria parasite's life cycle. The merozoite, trophozoite, schizont, and gametocyte are present in the red blood cells of the warm-blooded host. All, except the gametocyte, replicate by asexual reproduction. The gametocyte is the immature gamete.

Each stage is not only morphologically distinct but antigenically distinct as well. For example, if a vaccine were made from merozoites (the stage which invades red blood cells) it would not prevent acquiring the infection from a mosquito bite delivering the sporozoite stage (the infective stage present in the mosquito's salivary glands). Work has progressed rapidly in a variety of directions. One direction espoused by a coterie of malaria vaccinologists is to make a vaccine from sporozoites since this would prevent malaria in the first place—from the mosquito's bite. Previous research had already shown that living sporozoites attenuated for infectivity by irradiating them with X-ray or some other radioactive source induced immune protection in animals and in the few human volunteers in which this living vaccine had been injected. However, irradiated sporozoites are not a very practical proposition as a vaccine. For one thing, they are very hard to come by—they can't be "farmed" in test-tube culture; they must be obtained from the salivary glands of infected mosquitoes. And even if means were found to obtain large numbers of "clean" sporozoites it still wouldn't make for a practical vaccine since it would be virtually impossible to maintain them in a living state until they could be delivered to the tropical villages where they would be injected into the locals.

Research begun by the group at New York University's Department of Medical and Molecular Parasitology has circumvented the difficulties by identifying the immunizing antigenic determinant (epitope) on the sporozoite's surface and then synthesizing a man-made replica of it. That synthetic replica has afforded a high level of protection in animals and although it—and other synthetic candidate vaccines—are currently being tested for safety in human volunteers, the crucial experiment of giving a human being an immunizing course of injections followed by the challenging bites of infected mosquitoes has yet to be carried out.

As promising as all this is, there are problems associated with synthetic vaccines that have to be overcome if they are ever to be used on more than an experimental basis. Synthetic epitope vaccines, as I have already pointed out, require a carrier protein. There is still no carrier protein sufficiently free of adverse side effects that it would be approved by the FDA for use in humans. Furthermore, some synthetic vaccines do not induce enough immunity to afford protection. They can be antigens without being immunogens. These feeble vaccines need to be mixed with a strange conglomeration of substances called *adjuvants*. Adjuvants amplify the immune response brought forth by the antigen with which it is mixed. One author noted that the variety of adjuvants used reads like an alchemist's shopping list. Freund's adjuvant (a mixture of oil, water, and bacteria related to the *Mycobacterium* of tuberculosis), saponin (a product from the soapwort and other plants), alum, and vitamin A are few examples of adjuvant diversity. The eye of newt and its accompanying incantation has yet to be tried; it may turn out to be the best adjuvant of all. The trouble is that very few of the adjuvants have been approved for use in humans. However, the alchemist's shopping list keeps growing and some safe, potent adjuvants are expected on the scene within the next few years. There are a few synthetic vaccines that give indication of inducing a protective immunity without either a carrier protein or adjuvant. These undoubtedly are the synthetics that will be first used in man.

The crystal ball foretells that these new directions in vaccine development—the recombinant gene techniques and the synthesis of essential antigenic determinants—will permit us to immunize humans against diseases for which no vaccine is now available. The National Institutes of Health (the American flagship biomedical research institution) predicts that within the next ten years there will be new vaccines to immunize humans against chickenpox, genital herpes, malaria, gonorrhea, and croup in infants (respiratory syncytial virus). A large body of ongoing research is directed to spreading the vaccine net to even a larger diversity of infectious diseases and there are immunologists who foresee, in the not-too-distant future, vaccines to protect us against colds, leprosy, syphilis, viral gastroenteritis, bacterial meningitis, African sleeping sickness, blood flukes (schistosomes), and filarial worms (parasites that cause elephantiasis and river blindness).

There are also visionaries who maintain that the prevention of disease by immunization does not have to be limited to the infectious diseases. The great golden prize would be the development of vaccine(s) to protect us from cancer(s). The logic that gives substance to this dream is that when normal cells transform to precancerous or cancerous cells they acquire antigens which the body recognizes as foreign antigenic. Theoretically, given the appropriate techniques and immunizing strategies, at least some of these cancer-associated antigens can be exploited for vaccine development.

A step further back would be to immunize against the agents that induce cancers. Virus-induced cancers would be the most likely form of cancers amenable to this approach. There are two cancers of animals known to be caused by viruses: Marek's lymphoma in chickens, and feline leukemia in cats. It is almost (but not irrefutably) proven that a group of human cancers are also caused by oncogenic viruses;

the best case presently being for the Epstein-Barr virus as the causative agent of Burkitt's lymphoma. During the next twenty years other viruses will probably be be incriminated and a few others proven as being oncogenic in human cancers. When that research comes to fruition it should be possible, by one or more of the genetic engineering-synthetic techniques, to develop cancer-protecting vaccines from those viruses. Effective vaccines are already available to protect chickens against Marek's lymphoma and cats against feline leukemia. What we can do for chickens and cats we should be able to do for humans. A prediction: Some types of leukemia will be shown to have a viral etiology and sometime during the next century children will be immunized against leukemia with the ease and frequency as they are now immunized against polio. In the tropics, children will be vaccinated against Burkitt's lymphoma. In adults some cancers will be proven to have a viral etiology (colorectal cancers may be among that group) and protective vaccines will be developed.

The majority of cancers do not seem to be caused by viruses, however, and the actual direct or indirect causes for these "spontaneous" cancers may never be discovered. Will it ever be possible to vaccinate against these cancers? I wouldn't bet the family jewels on it, but I will predict that in time (and that time frame being unpredictable) some of those cancers will also become preventable by vaccination's immune protection.

For more than half a century, cancer researchers have been injecting mice and other experimental animals with a variety of preparations derived from cancer cells in attempts to induce a protective immunization. The results have been variable, but there have been sufficient successes to encourage the idea that immunization may be an attainable goal. Analogous experiments have not been carried out in humans. Humans haven't been given a series of injections with an extract of tumor cells and then their immunity put to the test by having the tumor implanted in them. Nor have large numbers of humans been given immunizing injections and then followed for twenty to fifty years to determine if the number of cases of cancer was significantly fewer in the immunized group than in the matched unimmunized control group.

What has been done in a limited number of human experiments is to inject patients already stricken with cancer with vaccines prepared from homologous cancers or preparations made from their own cancer cells. The objective of those trials was to invigorate specifically the patient's immune system to a degree that it would halt the progress of the disease and, at best, to bring about regression of tumor growth and cure. One such study, begun in the late 1970s, involved patients with lung cancer. Their cancers were, as far as it was possible, surgically removed. Half the patients were then given three monthly injections of a vaccine made from lung cancer cells along with a conventional course of postoperative chemotherapy. The other half of the patients were given the postoperative chemotherapy only. The vaccine immunotherapy had an effect but only when given to patients whose cancer, before surgery, was at an early stage of development (stage I). After four years, 83 percent of these patients were still alive, whereas for the stage-I cancer group that had been given postoperative chemotherapy alone the survival rate was 49 percent. The immunotherapy had no effect in extending the life of patients with more advanced cancers when they came to surgery. These were not dramatic results (except perhaps to that 34 percent who had been given a new lease on life) but it did indicate that even with what now seem crude vaccines, specific immunotherapy can play a role in the treatment of cancer providing that treatment is begun when the cancer is at an early stage.

In my overworked, clouded crystal ball I see vaccines, made by genetic engineering techniques, that are specific antigenic determinants expressed by cancer cells. It is unlikely that a "universal" vaccine to protect against all cancers will ever be found. Present indications would have it that each type of cancer is associated with antigens peculiar to it. Furthermore, anticancer immunizations will probably not be solidly protective, and freedom from cancer will come only when there is an accompanied change in life-style—such as renouncing tobacco and adopting a defensive anticancer diet. For the unfortunate who slip through these defenses and do acquire cancers, I predict that within the next twenty years there will be an immunotherapeutic package (more on this presently) of which immune therapy will be a component to replace or supplement drug therapy. The more vatic immunologists predict that the time will come when the immunotherapeutic means will be at hand to have the cancerous body cure itself.

## Anti-Baby Vaccines

Immunizations against pregnancy? Why not? Pregnancy is hardly a disease, but in its guise of uncontrolled population growth it is a blight on the world. While in Dacca last year I had dinner with the physician who is the U.S. Agency for International Development (AID) advisor to Bangladesh's family-planning program. "We did about forty-thousand tubal litigation sterilizations last month," he said. "That's great," I said. "Just about all of them were grandmothers," he said. "That's not so good." I said, "Why were they all so old?" "They weren't so old," he said. "Most were about thirty-five years old. They married when they were fourteen or fifteen, and when they finally decided to call it reproductively quits they already had had five or more children."

The conversation with my friend from AID illustrates a common problem in population control programs. Too many Third World women don't begin practicing birth control until they have too many babies. Men aren't all that reliable as the "controlled" partner. All men have is celibacy, condoms, and vasectomy. They may be persuaded to use the condom, but celibacy is contrary to psycho-hormonal drives, and vasectomy, for many men, is too threatening in a final-solution way. Nor do women—particularly the women of the Third World—have satisfactory birth-control methods even when they accept the idea that family size should be limited to one or two children. Sterilization is as traumatic to women as it is to men. Who wants to go under the knife? Especially if the operating room is a table in the village health center. Too many women refuse to take "the pill," or when they do take it, fail to comply to the regime. IUDs are apt to be uncomfortable, sometimes dangerous, and thus too often and too soon rejected as a form of birth control by the women in whom they have been inserted.

It is generally conceded that completely new, acceptable, and effective birth-control measures are needed if universal family-planning programs, free of coercion, are to succeed. An attractive, novel birth-control method would be to vaccinate against pregnancy. Experimental animals and, theoretically, humans can be made immune to pregnancy. The proteins, especially the proteins that determine histocompatibility (MHC) type that make a sperm a sperm, are foreign to a woman and are therefore potentially anti-genic. The fetus is even more massively antigenic. It would be immunologically correct to express your felicitations to the new mother with "Congratulations on the birth of your nine-pound foreign body." Half the MHC antigens of the embryo are contributed by Daddy. This makes the embryo, as far as the mother is concerned, as much of a parasite as a tapeworm, and as foreign as a skin graft from a total stranger. Sex is a wonderful thing—it defies the fundamen-tal (immunological) laws of nature. One of the major, unsolved immunological mysteries is how the mother can tolerate her cherished parasite without her body mounting an immune response to reject it. Experimentally, the uterus will reject a graft of tissue of different histocompatability type, so there is nothing unnaturally peculiar to it in the immunological sense. Several explanatory theories have been offered. One theory proposes that maternal hormones and suppressor T cells in the placenta inhibit the immune response on the part of the mother as well as on the part of the fetus (the immune system is formed quite early in fetal life—the fetus is immunocompetent by the third month of life, and thus, the fetus imaginably could reject the mother). Another theory that is currently favored by many immu-nologists is that the anatomical physical separation between mother and embryo effectively prevents severe immune stimuli and reactions.

Reproductive immunologists believe that with the right antigens it should be possible to upset this balanced, com-mensal-like relationship and to immunize women against pregnancy. This experimental game is barely afoot, but several antigens have been identified as to their antire-productive potential as immunogens. One of these antigens is oncofetal antigen. Oncofetal antigen is present in sperm and in the fetus during early embryonic life (it also becomes expressed by many types of cancer cells and is a diagnostic marker for these cancers). A vaccine made or derived from this antigen might, conceivably (inconceivably?), induce an immune status in the mother that would abort the pregnancy within a few days after conception.

Another possible means of antireproductive vaccination would employ a hormone as the antigen. As any pregnant mother knows, there are distinct hormonal changes during pregnancy: changes essential to maintaining that pregnancy. One participating hormone is known as human chorionic gonadotropin (HCG) and it is produced, not by the mother, but by the fetus. Immunologists have reasoned that if women could be vaccinated to produce specific anti-HCG antibodies, the antibodies would inactivate the hormone and the women in effect would be infertile. This is a very clever approach that hasn't come to fruition because the antibodies formed against HCG cross-react with other essential hormones, and this has an adverse effect on the normal sexual "tone" of the body. Expectations are that a highly specific epitope that will induce antibody completely specific to HCG will be "dissected" from the hormone's molecule. If and when that epitope is identified and can be linked to an acceptable protein carrier, antihormone vaccination could become an important strategy in population control.

To forestall the acid comments of my wife (the primary "stalking horse" reader of my draft manuscripts)—"Why must it always be the women? Why don't you men get vaccinated and become infertile?"—let me hasten to add that vaccination of men is being considered as a possible means of birth control. Although I think men would offer their arms to the vaccinator's needle, there are potential difficulties in making males infertile by immunological methods.

One of the strange things about men is that their own sperm is antigenically foreign to them: their immune system doesn't recognize the sperm as "self"—as a member of the body corporate. Fortunately, sperm are manufactured by, and discharged through, an anatomical construction that when normal and intact acts as a barrier (the blood-testis barrier) to the recognition-surveillance cells of the immune system. Where there is leakage across a defective barrier, antibodies (autoantibodies) and cellular reactions can occur to cause inflammatory, degenerative conditions of the sexual tract (orchitis, epididymitis). This has made investigators cautious in trying to devise a male birth-control vaccine. The trick would be to find a sperm antigen that would induce antibody formation without the risk of causing an associated autoimmune disease—the kind of immune state that occurs in most men after vasectomy.[9] Antibody-coated sperm lose that vigorous wiggle, that dance of life, needed to insinuate their way through the cervical mucus to get to the egg.

It is possible that a male birth-control vaccine would not be derived from human sperm. In 1980, two scientists, A. Lopo and V. D. Vacquier, reported in *Nature* that when they vaccinated rabbits with the sperm of a sea urchin the antibody elicited not only inactivated sea-urchin sperm but cross-reacted to "de-fertilize" human sperm as well. They

9. One of the most common ways that the blood-testis barrier becomes compromised and antibodies to sperm develop is from vasectomy. Most vasectomized men have anti-sperm antibodies. Fortunately, there is no convincing evidence that this leads to autoimmune disease.Why the immune reaction as a consequence of vasectomy is essentially benign and the immune reaction to other forms of self-immunization to sperm are potentially pathogenic is not known.

suggested that sea-urchin sperm, especially the immuogenic component of their sperm, could serve as a suitable vaccine for birth control. Wouldn't it be strangely unexpected if one of the world's thorniest human problems was solved with this lowly, prickly creature?

## Immune Targeting: Delivering the Goods with Monoclonals

Astronauts, archers, and artillerymen who arrive on target with high precision would be appalled by the manner in which therapeutic agents are sent to their destinations. Taking most drugs is much like casting a stone into the still waters of a pond. The drug is absorbed into the bloodstream and diffuses through the body like the ripples radiating across the pond's surface. Therapeutic agents are thus effective only when they are potent enough to exert their activity at the low concentrations of random dilution. The archives of pharmacological research are voluminous with drugs that showed great promise but couldn't cut the mustard because of their inability to be where they were needed in the body at effective concentration. And most drugs are poisons; they kill the pathogenic cell and microorganism or reform the defectively functioning cell by altering essential biochemical processes. For the most part, the pathogen and the normal cell of the body have a basic common chemistry. The metabolism of the abnormal cell and pathogen is subtly different and the drug acts selectively on them. That is, it acts selectively but not exclusively: the normal cell is "poisoned" also, but at a sufficiently low level as to make the drug tolerable.

The problem that has vexed physicians and pharmacologists is how to direct the drug to the focus where it is needed. The chemotherapy of cancer has been especially hampered by this limitation because anticancer drugs tend to be highly toxic. There have been a number of inventive delivery modes devised, such as implanting a drug reservoir and miniaturized pump in the site of the affected organ, but none have been entirely successful. The introduction of hybridoma technology for monoclonal antibody production gives promise that an unerringly targeted delivery system is within our grasp.

The idea that antibodies can deliver the goods is not new. In 1906, the Wizard of Silesia, Paul Ehrlich, proposed that toxins and drugs could be conjugated to a specific antibody and sent to the cells which elicited the antibody. A sound idea that has, until recent years, been confounded by the limitations of experimentally produced antibodies. Try as they might by antigen purification and repeated immunizations, immunologists could not obtain antibodies that were specifically pure or potent enough to be used as a carrier. Even under the most exacting experimental conditions the amount of specific antibody that could be obtained from an immunized animal was not more than 5 percent of the total serum immunoglobulins.

The advent of hybridoma technology for monoclonal antibody production has, theoretically, raised those restrictions. With monoclonal antibodies as carriers it is within the realm of possibility to: (1) identify the antigenic determinant (epitope) unique to the target cell; (2) produce absolutely specific antibody of a single immunoglobulin class, in unlimited quantities, to that epitope; and (3) conjugate a chemotherapeutic agent, toxin, or biologic immune modulator to the monoclonal that would then selectively deliver the therapeutic to the target cells as well as exert a synergistic antibody action on those cells.

Monoclonal antibodies are among modern immunology's most powerful and useful tools. Before I make any more promises let me take a narrative moment to describe what they are and what they do. E Pluribus Immunity has it that there are at least 100 million different epitopes, and for each epitope there is a waiting companion B cell that can be transformed to become an expanded clone of antibody-secreting plasma cells. If a laboratory animal were injected with a "crude" mixture of antigens—ground-up whole bacteria, for example—many clones of plasma cells would be present in its spleen. Immunologists need absolutely "pure" antibody (specific for a single epitope) for their research, and this could theoretically be obtained by taking the plasma cells from the spleen of an immunized animal and isolating them as single cells in culture medium. One plasma cell = one antibody. At this point, technology ground to a halt. The plasma cell couldn't be persuaded to divide perpetually in culture (to form an expanded clone) from which the antibody could be harvested. Plasma cells in both the body and the culture have a short life span and a limited reproductive capacity. However, this reproductive limit is removed when the plasma cell becomes cancerous.

Like other cell types of the body, the plasma cell can be transformed to become cancerous (a plasma cell cancer is called a *myeloma*). When cells become cancerous or pre-cancerous, they also become immortal. They will divide forever in the test tube, and in the body, given the chance (except that the body is vulnerably mortal and dies from the selfish cancer's desire for everlasting life).

In 1975, two immunologists, G. Kohler and C. Milstein, devised a technique to fuse a normal, antibody-secreting plasma cell to a cancerous plasma (myeloma) cell. They named this immunological centaur a *hybridoma*. The

hybridoma was immortal, like the myeloma cell component, but secreted the specific antibody of its plasma cell
partner. The method for making hybridomas results in a
suspension of thousands of fused (hybridoma) cells, each
one capable of secreting its own unique antibody. The
painstaking task is to select the hybridoma that is elaborating the antibody of the desired specificity. To do this, each
hybridoma cell is isolated and placed by itself in a tube
containing a suitable culture medium. Under these conditions, the hybridoma cell will multiply to form an antibody
secreting tumor mass. The antibody, now in the culture
medium, is collected and analyzed for its specificity. With
a bit of care and lots of luck the desired hybridoma is in
one of those tubes. This clone line can then be expanded
for large-scale *monoclonal antibody* production ("monoclonal" because it originates from a single plasma cell
hybridoma and has a single epitopic specificity). Alterna-
tively, the cells of the selected hybridoma can be inoculated into the abdominal cavity of a mouse, where they will
grow into a monoclonal antibody–secreting tumor. While
the mouse lives, its ascitic fluid—which contains a high
concentration of antibody—can be collected and purified
for experimental, therapeutic, and diagnostic uses.

Monoclonal-carrier targeting to cancers has been a major
objective of this still very new field of research. Most of the
investigations have centered on mouse cancers, because
many of the antigens of murine (mouse) cancers are known
and because there also exists a sizeable hybridoma "library"
to them. Also, the great majority of monoclonals are of mouse
hybridoma origin, so there is no problem (as there is in
humans—as I shall note shortly) of untoward sensitization
to the antibody carrier. Here again the ghost of Paul Ehrlich walks. Among the initial candidate agents considered

for conjugation were the plant toxins ricin and abrin, the toxins Ehrlich used to demonstrate the principle of antibody specifity. The plant toxins and the incredibly lethal bacterial toxins (such as the botulism toxin) act by inhibiting protein thesis. They are, thus, overwhelmingly poisonous to rapidly dividing cells. Cancer cells are an example par excellence of cells undergoing rapid, unrestrained division. But the toxins are toxic for normal cells as well. With toxins conjugated to monoclonal antibodies specific for cancer antigens it has been possible to confine their toxic activity to cancer cells only. In these experiments the normal cells of the body were spared and several murine cancers cured. Anticancer drugs such as cyclophosphamide and anticancer antibiotics such as adriamycin have been similarly linked to mouse anticancer monoclonal antibodies and delivered to tumors to produce high, localized concentrations of drug.

Virus-infected cells that acquire specific antigens on their outer membrane have been similarly targeted with an assortment of antiviral agents conjugated to monoclonals.

Immune troubles? Too many suppressor cells—as occurs in AIDS and rheumatoid arthritis—and insufficient immunoglobulin production? Suppressor T cells have their own characteristic antigen markers to which monoclonal antibodies have been made. It should be possible to send these monoclonals, linked to a lymphotoxic agent, to knock them out and redress the abnormal helper T cell–suppressor T cell balance. Similarly, helper-cytotoxic T cells could be knocked off to inhibit organ transplant rejection.

Regrettably, it will be some years before you can go to your doctor for an injection of this new kind of monoclonal "magic bullet." A major problem, as I have briefly noted, is that the vast majority of hybridomas are formed from mouse myeloma cells fused to mouse plasma cells. Although the monoclonal antibody produced by these hybridomas may be directed against antigenic determinants of human origin they are, nevertheless, mouse immunoglobulins that the human would recognize as foreign and elicit an antibody response. Thus, more than one injection of a mouse-derived monoclonal could result in a massively adverse antigen-antibody reaction so severe in its shock-like effect as to be fatal. One possible dodge is to use only the "V"—the Fab portion—of the total (Y) monoclonal immunoglobulin molecule. It is that portion, you will recall, that bears the complimentary receptor (idiotope) that "docks" with the antigen determinant (epitope). Unfortunately, for some unknown reason, Fabs act less well in an immune response than do intact immunoglobulins. Also for some unknown reason, Fabs do not adhere to the antigen with the same tenacity as do intact immunoglobulin molecules, and the drug conjugated to the Fab monoclonal tends to dissociate from the target cell before the drug can do its work.

The ideal would be to use hybridomas from human cells. Those hybridomas would elaborate "antigenically human" monoclonal antibodies that could be safely used to treat humans. The technology to make human hybridomas has been developed only during these past few years, and it is still to be perfected. The "library" of human monoclonal antibodies is at present modestly small, but it will grow, and monoclonal antibodies will become drug-carrying missiles. The crystal ball reveals a clear picture of the monoclonal antibody in our therapeutic future.

"Promises, promises" is not immunology's bombast. There are not many biomedical sciences that promise so much with the same expectation of fulfillment. Immunology has an almost unrivalled vitality that I would liken to a great Eastern bazaar—buoyantly thriving, filled with gems and baubles, wheeling and dealing. A few weeks ago during a coffee-break conversation with some visitors and colleagues I imagined I was back in the Souk of Istanbul.

VISITOR A. The malaria vaccine is a success!

AUTHOR. Success? You haven't gotten around to protecting anything more than monkeys—and they haven't been immunized all *that* successfully?

VISITOR A. Listen, I'm getting a million dollars for vaccine research. If that isn't a success I don't know what is.

COLLEAGUE A. That million won't do you any good. You're too late in the race. We're making synthetic vaccines from scratch—right out of the bottle. We are going to fabricate the vaccine as soon as the chemical design is worked out.

COLLEAGUE B (a molecular biologist). That's no great accomplishment. For a billion dollars I can make, and put into place, the genes that would make the immune response so efficient that a vaccine won't be necessary.

VISITOR B (another molecular biologist). And for two billion dollars I can create the genes to create a human that goes with that designer-gened immune system.

And why not? It's only money.

# Index